Recent Developments in Graves' Ophthalmopathy

Recent Developments in Graves' Ophthalmopathy

edited by

Mark F. Prummel
Academic Medical Center
Amsterdam, The Netherlands

Co-Editors

Wilmar M. Wiersinga
Academic Medical Center
Amsterdam, The Netherlands

Maarten Ph. Mourits
University Medical Center
Utrecht, The Netherlands

Armin E. Heufelder
Philipps-Universität Marburg
Marburg, Germany

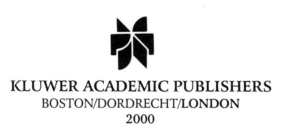

KLUWER ACADEMIC PUBLISHERS
BOSTON/DORDRECHT/LONDON
2000

Distributors for North, Central and South America:
Kluwer Academic Publishers
101 Philip Drive
Assinippi Park
Norwell, Massachusetts 02061 USA
Telephone (781) 871-6600
Fax (781) 871-6528
E-Mail <kluwer@wkap.com>

Distributors for all other countries:
Kluwer Academic Publishers Group
Distribution Centre
Post Office Box 322
3300 AH Dordrecht, THE NETHERLANDS
Telephone 31 78 6392 392
Fax 31 78 6546 474
E-Mail <services@wkap.nl>

Electronic Services <http://www.wkap.nl>

Library of Congress Cataloging-in-Publication Data

Recent developments in Graves' ophthalmopathy / edited by Mark F. Prummel;
co-editors, Wilmar M. Wiersinga, Maarten Ph. Mourits, Armin E. Heufelder.
     p. ; cm
  Includes bibliographical references and index.
  ISBN 0-7923-8676-0 (alk. paper)
  1.Thyroid eye disease. I. Prummel, Mark F.
  [DNLM: 1. Graves' Disease--therapy. 2. Graves' Disease--pathology. 3. Orbit--surgery.
WK 265 R295 2000]
RE715.T48 R434 2000
617.7--dc21

                        99-046681

Contents

Contributors

Rebecca S. BAHN, M.D., Ph.D., Professor of Endocrinology, Mayo Clinic Rochester, 200 First Street Southwest, Rochester, Minnesota 55905, United States of America.

Hemmo A. DREXHAGE, M.D., Ph.D., Professor of Immunology, Department of Immunology, Erasmus University Rotterdam, PO Box 1738, 3000 DR Rotterdam, The Netherlands

Steven E. FELDON, M.D., Ph.D., Professor of Ophthalmology, Neuro-ophthalmology/Oculoplastic Service, Doheny Eye Institute, 1355 San Pablo street, Los Angeles, California 90033, United States of America

James GARRITY, M.D., Ph.D., Professor of Ophthalmology, Department of Ophthalmology, Mayo Clinic Rochester, 200 First Street Southwest, Rochester, Minnesota 55905, United States of America.

Colum A. GORMAN, M.D., Ph.D., Professor of Endocrinology, Mayo Clinic Rochester, 200 First Street Southwest, Rochester, Minnesota 55905, United States of America.

Armin E. HEUFELDER, M.D., Ph.D., Professor of Endocrinology, Klinikum der Philipps-Universität Marburg, Zentrum für Innere Medizin, Abteilung Innere Medizin mit Schwerpunkt Gastroenterologie, Endokrinologie, Diabetologie; Baklingerstrasse, 35033-Marburg, Germany

George J. KAHALY, M.D., Ph.D., Professor of Endocrinology, Department of Endocrinology/Metabolism, Building 303, Johannes Gutenberg Klinikum, University of Mainz, 55101 Germany

Henk B. KAL, Ph.D., Netherlands Organization for Applied Scientific Research (TNO), Lange Kleiweg 151, P.O. Box, 2280 HV, Rijswijk, The Netherlands

Leo KOORNNEEF, M.D., Ph.D., Professor of Ophthalmology, Orbital Center, A2, Academic Medical Center, University of Amsterdam, Meibergdreef 9, 1105 AZ Amsterdam, The Netherlands

Marian LUDGATE, Ph.D., Department of Pathology, University of Wales College of Medicine, Heath Park, Cardiff CF4 4XN, United Kingdom

Claudio MARCOCCI, M.D., Ph.D., Department of Endocrinology, University of Pisa, Via Paradisa 2, 56124 Pisa, Italy

Guido MATTON, M.D., Ph.D., Professor of Surgery, Department of Plastic Surgery, University of Gent, University Hospital, De Pintelaan 185, B-9000 Gent, Belgium

Maarten Ph. MOURITS, M.D., Ph.D., Department of Ophthalmology, Orbital Center, University Medical Center Utrecht, Heidelberglaan 100, The Netherlands

Marco NARDI, M.D., Ph.D., Professor of Ophthalmology, Department of Neurosciences, Section of Ophthalmology, University of Pisa, Via Roma 67, 56126 Pisa, Italy

Aldo PINCHERA, M.D., Ph.D., Professor of Endocrinology, Department of Endocrinology, University of Pisa, Via Paradisa 2, 56124 Pisa, Italy

Mark F. PRUMMEL, M.D., Ph.D., Department of Endocrinology, Academic Medical Center, University of Amsterdam, Meibergdreef 9, 1105 AZ Amsterdam, The Netherlands

Geoffry E. ROSE, M.D., Ph.D.,MRCP, FRCS, FRCOphth., Consultant Ophthalmic Surgeon, Private Patients' Suite, Moorfields Eye Hospital, City Road, London EC1V 2PD, United Kingdom

H. Stevie TAN, M.D., Ph.D., Department of Ophthalmology, Academic Medical Center, University of Amsterdam, Meibergdreef 9, 1105 AZ Amsterdam, The Netherlands

Caroline B. TERWEE, M.Sc., Department of Clinical Epidemiology and Biostatistics, Academic Medical Center, University of Amsterdam, Meibergdreef 9, 1105 AZ Amsterdam, The Netherlands

Wilmar M. WIERSINGA, M.D., Ph.D., Professor of Endocrinology, Department of Endocrinology, Academic Medical Center, University of Amsterdam, Meibergdreef 9, 1105 AZ Amsterdam, The Netherlands

Anthony P. WEETMAN, M.D., Ph.D., Professor of Medicine, Division of Clinical Sciences, Northern General Hospital, The University of Sheffield, Herries Road, Sheffield S5 7AU, United Kingdom

Preface

Graves' ophthalmopathy is one of the most enigmatic and intriguing autoimmune disorders. It mesmerizes basic researchers, internists, and ophthalmologists alike, whereas it is appalling to the patient. For these reasons it is understandable that many meetings have been convened. Because of the variety of disciplines involved, joint meetings with orbital surgeons, endocrinologists, and immunologists have been the most informative.

Such joint conferences have been held in Montreal (1988), Amsterdam (1991), Rochester, Minnesota (1992), Mainz (1992), and Pittsburgh, Pennsylvania (1995). In November 1998 the VIth International Symposium on Graves' ophthalmopathy was held in Amsterdam, The Netherlands. Over 200 participants shared their knowledge and experience, and almost all experts in the field were present. This meeting inspired us to write this book. It aspires to not only summarize the most recent developments, but also to serve as a reference book, for all those who are puzzled by this always disfiguring and often invalidating disease. The disorder certainly needs a VIIth International Symposium.

Mark F. Prummel

Amsterdam, Summer

Recent Developments in
Graves' Ophthalmopathy

Chapter 1

Introduction to Graves' ophthalmopathy

Mark F. Prummel*, Leo Koornneef, Maarten Ph. Mourits, Armin E. Heufelder, Wilmar M. Wiersinga.
*Department of Endocrinology, Academic Medical Center, University of Amsterdam, Meibergdreef 9, 1105 AZ Amsterdam, The Netherlands

Although the pathogenesis of Graves' ophthalmopathy is incompletely understood, we have a rather good insight as to how the pathologic changes in the orbit cause (in a mechanical way) the clinical characteristics. To better understand this it is important to be acquainted with the anatomy of the orbit.

1.   ANATOMY OF THE ORBIT

The cavity containing the orbital tissues is completely surrounded by seven bones, except for the frontal opening where the globe is situated. Its shape is pear-like, and its axis directs backwards and medially (Fig. 1).[1]

The most anterior parts of the bones surrounding the orbital cavity form the orbital rim. The width of the opening is approximately 4 cm, the height 3.5 cm; the volume of the orbital cavity is appr. 30 ml. The medial walls run parallel, separated from each other by the paired ethmoid cells. The lateral walls form a 45 degree angle to their corresponding medial walls.

The roof of the orbit consists of the frontal bone and the lesser wing of the sfenoid, separating the brain from the orbit. The anterior medial part of the roof contains the frontal sinus, which dimensions vary considerably. The medial wall consists of the ethmoid bone with its very thin lamina papyracea, separating the orbit from the air-containing ethmoidal sinus. The medial wall further consists of the lacrimal bone, the lesser wing of the sfenoid bone and the tip of the maxilla. The floor is formed by the maxillary, palatine, and zygomatic bones and thus also forms the roof of the maxillary sinus.

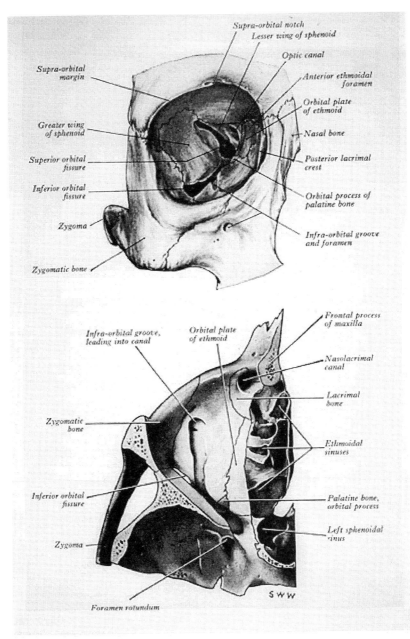

Figure 1. Upper panel: The right orbit, anterior aspect. Lower panel: A horizontal section through the left orbit and nasal cavity. Superior aspect. (reproduced with permission from the Publisher.[1])

The part of the floor medial to the infraorbital neurovascular bundle, which runs through a canal within the orbital floor, is thin; lateral to the nerve the floor is much thicker. At the anterior medial corner of the floor, the lacrimal fossa contains the lacrimal sac which is connected with the nasal cavity via the nasolacrimal duct. The lateral wall is the strongest and is composed of the greater wing of the sfenoid bone and of the zygomatic bone, separating the orbit from the infratemporal fossa. The orbital cavity is limited anteriorly by the orbital septum, which originates from the orbital rim and inserts onto the eyelid retractors. The orbit is lined with periorbita, which is part of an extremely well organized musculo-fibrous skeleton embedding the globe, the extraocular muscles, the optic nerve, vessels and other nerves, the laterosuperiorly localized lacrimal gland and orbital fat (Fig. 2). The globe itself is surrounded by a fascial sheath (Tenon's capsule), which fuses posteriorly with the optic nerve sheath.

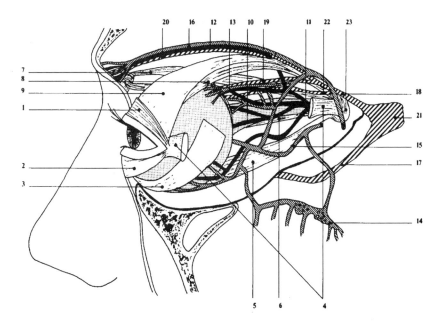

Figure 2. Schematic drawing of the orbital contents. 1, superior tarsal plate; 2, inferior tarsal plate; 3, inferior oblique muscle; 4, lateral rectus muscle (partly removed); 5, inferior rectus muscle; 6, medial rectus muscle; 7, superior oblique muscle; 8, superior rectus muscle; 9, levator palpebrae superioris muscle; 10, posterior ciliary arteries; 11, ophthalmic artery; 12, supraorbital artery; 13, dorsal nasal artery; pterygoid venous network; 15, inferior ophthalmic vein; 16, superior ophthalmic vein; 17, maxilla nerve; 18, ophthalmic nerve; 19, lacrimal nerve; 20 frontal nerve; 21, trigeminal ganglion; 22, nasocilliary nerve; 23, Zinn's annulus. (Reproduced with permission from the publisher.[29])

1.1   The Extraocular eye muscles (EOM)

There are seven EOM: four rectus muscles, two oblique muscles, and the levator palpebrae superioris (Fig. 2). Except for the latter, which moves the upper eye lid, the EOM are responsible for the movements of the eye ball. The superior levator muscle lifts the upper eye lid and is difficult to distinguish from the superior rectus muscle on imaging techniques. The anterior lamella consists of different layers radiating into the orbicularis muscle creating the skin crease. The posterior lamella consists of nonstriated muscle fibers forming the superior tarsal muscle. Both upper and lower eye lids contain nonstriated muscles and are innervated sympathetically. The other EOM are striated muscles, from mesodermal origin but originating from different myotomes as compared to the other (limb) skeletal muscles.[2] The four rectus muscles and the superior oblique muscle originate posteriorly from a tight fibrous ring (Zinn's annulus) around the optic nerve (Fig. 3). The inferior oblique arises from the periosteum of the medial part of the orbital floor at the lacrimal duct opening, the levator palpebrae arises from the sfenoid just outside the annulus of Zinn.

The rectus muscles are approximately 4 cm long and have to perforate Tenon's capsule before they reach the globe. Their tendons are of varying lengths and form the spiral of Tillaux, with the medial rectus having the shortest distance to the limbus and the superior rectus the longest. The superior oblique reaches the globe after passing through the trochlea, a cartilagineous structure near the medial part of the superior orbital rim. The upper eyelid retractor, e.g. the levator palpebrae is of special importance, because of its relationship with upper lid retraction. It is innervated by the superior branch of the oculomotor nerve and its aponeurosis passes downward from Whitnall's ligament and inserts onto the tarsus. On its posterior surface originates near Whitnall's ligament the sympathetic innervated Müller's muscle, which also inserts to the tarsus. Whitnall's ligament is part of the suspensory skeleton of the orbit.

The EOM are in some way different from other skeletal muscles. There are distinct ultrastructural differences with the limb muscles,[3] and the EOM have more variation in fiber size and type.[4] The fibers are arranged in two concentric zones with ill defined boundaries: an outer orbital layer adjacent to the periorbita, and an inner global layer adjacent to the optic nerve and eye ball.[2,4] The orbital layer consists of two types: the orbital singly innervated, and the orbital multiply innervated fibers. The global layer consists of four fiber subtypes (global red singly innervated fibers, global intermediate singly innervated fibers, global pale singly innervated fibers, and the global multiply innervated fibers). Thus the EOM are different from the other limb skeletal muscles, and in some ways are more comparable to amphibian muscles.[4] Apart from these morphological differences, they also contain different isoforms of myosin heavy chains.[5,6] First, EOM are different from limb muscles in that they continue to express embryonic myosin isoforms. Secondly, various myosin isoforms are present in the same fibers, and thirdly, EOM express myosin isoforms not present in other skeletal muscles.[4]

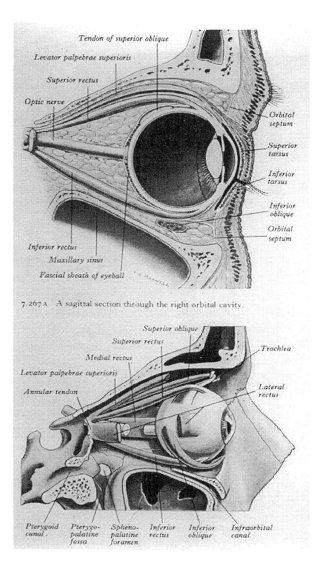

Figure 3. Upper panel: A sagittal section through the right orbital cavity. Lower panel: The muscles of the right orbit. Lateral aspect. (Reproduced with permission from the Publisher.[1])

1.2   Adipose and connective tissue.

The EOM are embedded in a well developed connective tissue network that interconnects the muscles and is attached to the periorbita.[7] This connective tissue forms multiple septa which are involved in the normal eye movements (Fig. 4).[8]

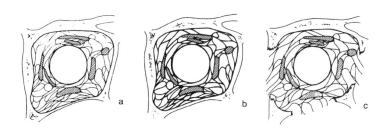

Figure 4. Schematic drawing of a coronal, histological section of the intraorbital connective tissue. A, normal connective tissue at eye ball level; b, hypertrophied connective tissue of a Graves' ophthalmopathy patient, explaining the enhancement seen on CT-scan. Note the relative increase in the number of septal connections with the periorbita near the orbital floor explaining the restriction in elevation; c, post decompression situation with the liberation of the pathologic and fibrotic bonds. (Reproduced with permission from the Publisher.[29])

The EOM and these septa are surrounded by a large quantity of adipose tissue. The orbit with its volume of 26 ml contains 18.9 g of retrobulbar tissue of which 63% is fat (12 g). The EOM only weigh 3.3 g (17%), the lacrimal gland 0.65 g, the rest being tendons, vessels and nerves.[9] The anatomy of the blood vessels has recently been characterized elegantly using MRI.[10] The orbit is vascularized by the ophthalmic artery, which extensively anastomizes with the external carotid circulation, for example by the anterior and posterior ethmoid arteries, that enter the orbit through openings in the medial wall at the frontoethmoidal suture. Angular, nasofrontal and supra-orbital veins drain posteriorly via the superior orbital vein on the cavernous sinus. No lymphatics draining the orbit have been detected. However, immunocompetent cells have been found consistently in the EOM, and the connective tissue and adipose tissues.[11,12] They are mainly T-suppressor cells and macrophages, which are heterogeneous and include dendritic cells capable of antigen presentation.[13]

The optic nerve is 4.5 -5.0 cm long and has an intraocular segment, an intraorbital part which is S-shaped, an intracanalicular and an intracranial segment. The optic nerve is covered with pia, arachnoidea and dura and the intracranial subarachnoid space communicates with that around the optic nerve. Two sensory nerves are of special interest. The supraorbital nerve, which branches from the frontal nerve, enters through an incisura or foramen in the superior rim and supplies the skin of the ipsilateral forehead. It should be chiseled out of its bony canal in coronal orbital approaches. The infraorbital nerve, which is often involved in orbital floor fractures, runs through a canal in the orbital floor, passes through the infraorbital foramen and supplies the ipsilateral skin of the cheek and upper lip.

2.   PATHOLOGY

The most prominent finding in GO is swelling of the EOM which can become grossly enlarged. For example, Rundle *et al.*[14] weighted the EOM of a 69 years old male with very severe GO since April 1952, who died form a myocardial infarction November 1952. His six EOM had all swollen to a similar degree, including the levator palpebrae (Table 1). The swollen muscles felt rubber-like and some had a diameter of >1 cm. On microscopy the muscles showed fibrosis, edema, and lymphocytic infiltration. The swelling of the muscles was not due to an increase in the number of fibers, but due to an increase in the volume of the individual fibers plus an increase in connective tissue. The water content of the adipose tissue was increased, but in this case the authors did not observe an increase in fatty tissue weight. In their earlier series in patients with GO who died in the thyrotoxic state, they did find such an increase in adipose tissue.[9]

Table 1. Weights of the extraocular eye muscles (mean of right and left orbit) in a 63 yr. old male with malignant GO of recent onset, who died from a myocardial infarction. Weights are compared to the mean weights found in 29 controls.[14]

Muscles	weight (g)	mean ±SD weight in 29 controls	Fold increase in weight vs. controls
Superior rectus	2.20	0.49 ±0.06	4.9
Medial rectus	3.41	0.87 ± 0.11	3.8
Inferior rectus	2.86	0.66 ± 0.08	4.2
Lateral rectus	2.17	0.72 ± 0.10	3.3
Superior oblique	0.68	0.27 ± 0.01	2.8
Levator palpebrae	1.46	0.41 ± 0.06	3.7

The inferior oblique muscle was not accessible for evaluation.

There is no consensus as to whether the adipose tissue compartment is swollen in Graves' ophthalmopathy. Both Feldon *et al.*,[15] and Trokel *et al.*[16] could not detect a significant increase in adipose tissue volume on CT-scan. On the other hand using three-dimensional volumetric CT-scans, van der Gaag *et al.*[17] found swelling of the EOM alone in 20% of their 40 GO patients. In 48% both the EOM and the adipose tissues were swollen, whereas in 28% the EOM volume was normal but the adipose tissue compartment had increased in volume; in 4 % no increase in orbital tissues was apparent. Using a similar technique, Forbes *et al.*[18] reached the same conclusions. It therefore appears that muscles, fat as well as the lacrimal gland, all can increase considerably in volume.

Already in the earliest descriptions it was noted that this swelling is due to an increase in what was called ground-substance. Now we know that this consists of collagen and glycosaminoglycans (GAG), which can be found throughout the muscle fibers in the endomysial space.[19] The GAG most prominently present is hyaluronan.[19] Despite this accumulation of GAG's and collagen between the muscle fibers, there is no evidence for ultrastructural damage to the EOM cells themselves. The sarcomeric organization remains intact,[20] and electron microscopy has not revealed any subcellular damage.[21] In addition to these depositions, many authors have found an increased amount of fibroblasts within endomyseal space and in the connective/adipose tissues. These infiltrating fibroblasts are considered to be the cells responsible for the overproduction of GAG's. GAG's are hydrophilic and can thus attract water and cause edema of the eye muscles and other affected retrobulbar tissues. Apart from these fibroblasts, there is also a mononuclear cell infiltration, consisting of lymphocytes, macrophages, and plasmacells. The nature of this infiltrate will be discussed in Chapter 2.

Thus the main pathology is an increase in the volume of all retrobulbar tissues. At autopsy, several investigators have noted that upon opening the periorbita, the accumulated adipose tissue promptly prolapses into the incision.[14,21] This suggests that apart from the increase in volume, there is also an increase in retrobulbar pressure, at least in severe cases. This, indeed, appears to be true. Otto validated an intraorbitally positioned micro-pressure transducer to measure the retrobulbar pressure in monkeys. He used this method in GO patients who were decompressed surgically.[22] In eight orbits with 'malignant' ophthalmopathy (e.g. sight loss due to optic nerve involvement), the retrobulbar pressure ranged from 17-40 mmHg (mean: 29 mmHg), and fell upon decompression by 9-12 mmHg. In contrast in two patients decompressed because of rehabilitative reasons, the retrobulbar pressure was only 9 and 11 mmHg, and did not change after the decompression, which was successful in terms of proptosis reduction.

3.   CLINICAL CHARACTERISTICS

With knowledge of the pathology of GO it is now easier to understand how the plethora of signs and symptoms in these patients occur. The main clinical features are summarized in the Werner Classification, known as NOSPECS (Table 2).[23]

Class 1. Only signs, no symptoms. This refers to the upper eyelid retraction frequently observed in patients with Graves' thyroid disease. This retraction causes stare, and lid lag on downward gaze (Von Graefe's sign) and can be due to swelling of the superior levator muscle. However, thyrotoxicosis per se can also induce this sign by increasing the sympathetic tone, and Von Graefe's sign is sometimes also present in hyperthyroidism not caused by Graves' disease.[24] Sympathetic overactivity is not the only cause of lid retraction, because overactivity of the *intra ocular* muscles (causing slower accommodation due to an increase in sympathetic tone) was shown to be unrelated to the presence or absence of upper eyelid retraction.[25] Therefore, it is likely that eyelid retraction is multifactorial in origin and it might well be that adhesions around the superior levator are another cause of retraction.[26] This would explain why upper eye lid retraction frequently remains present when GO patients are rendered euthyroid.

Class 2. Soft tissue involvement. This entails chemosis (edema of the conjunctiva), conjunctival injection and redness, and swollen upper and lower eyelids. These findings are partly explained by an impaired venous drainage as a result of the increase in retrobulbar tissue. This cannot be the only reason, because retrobulbar pressure is probably not always elevated, the removal rate of retro-bulbarly injected labeled fluid was found to be normal,[27] and soft tissue swelling usually remains after decompressive surgery. Another explanation for the swelling of the eyelids is herniation of retrobulbar tissue through the naturally occurring herniations in the orbital septum.[28,29]

Class 3. Proptosis. Because of the confining bony surroundings, the swollen retrobulbar tissue have no other outlet than pushing the globe forward. Hence, exophthalmos has even been termed 'nature's own decompression'.[30] In their meticulous postmortem studies Rundle and Pochin demonstrated that the normal orbital volume of the eye muscles is about 3.5 ml and that of the orbital cavity 26 ml.[9] They then showed that an increase in muscle volume of 4 ml causes a proptosis of 6 mm. Thus, small changes in tissue volume can cause considerable proptosis.

Class 4. Extraocular muscle involvement. One can easily imagine that swelling of the normally thin (Fig. 5) EOM leads to impaired mobility. If impairment is asymmetrical, the patient will have double vision. It is important to realize that the diplopia is of a binocular nature: if impairment is exactly symmetrical, or has become so by adapting the head position (ocular torticollis), there will be no diplopia. The same will occur, if the visual acuity in one eye is low, like in amblyopia.

Table 2. Classification of Eye Changes of Graves' ophthalmopathy: The NO SPECS classification.[23]

Class	Grade	Suggestions for grading
0		*N*o physical signs or symptoms
1		*O*nly signs
2		*S*oft tissue involvement
	0	Absent
	a	Minimal
	b	Moderate
	c	Marked
3		*P*roptosis 3 mm or more above upper normal limit; grading for Caucasian race
	0	Absent
	a	23-24 mm
	b	25-27 mm
	c	≥28 mm
4		*E*xtraocular muscle involvement: graded according to diplopia
	0	Absent
	a	Intermittent (when fatigued)
	b	Inconstant (at extremes of gaze)
	c	Constant (in primary gaze)
5		*C*orneal Involvement
	0	Absent
	a	Stippling of cornea
	b	Ulceration
	c	Clouding, necrosis, perforation
6		*S*ight loss due to optic nerve involvement
	0	Absent, vision ≥0.8
	a	Disc pallor, visual field defect, vision 0.63-0.5
	b	Same, but vision 0.4-0.1
	c	Same, but vision <0.1-blindness

For a long time, the diplopia was ascribed to paresis of one or more of the EOM, hence the term 'ophthalmoplegia'. However, we now know that the mobility impairment is caused by restricted relaxation of the affected antagonist. This can be appreciated by the 'forced duction test'. By actually grasping the globe and attempting to move it in the affected direction, mechanical resistance is felt.[31]

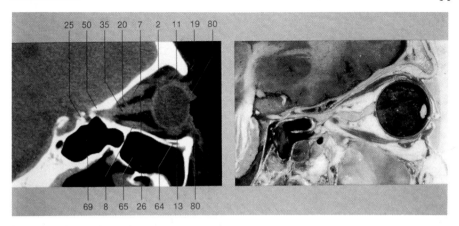

Figure 5a. CT section and cryosection in the sagital plane. 2, vitreous body; 7, superior rectus muscle complex; 8, inferior rectus muscle; 11, superior oblique tendon; 13, inferior oblique muscle; 19, orbicularis muscle; 20, ophthalmic artery; 25, internal carotid artery; 26, superior ophthalmic vein; 35, optic nerve; 50, lesser wing of the sphenoid bone; 64, infraorbital canal; 65, maxillary sinus; 69, sphenoidal sinus; 80, eye lid. (Reproduced with permission from the Publisher, Philips Medical Systems Division, Eindhoven, The Netherlands)

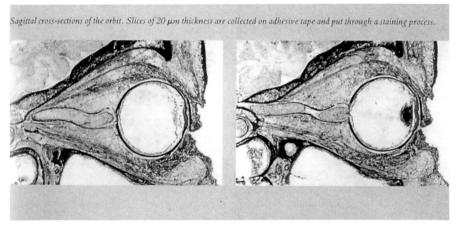

Figure 5b. Sagittal cross-sections of the orbit. Slices of 20 μm thickness collected on adhesive tape and put through a staining process. Note the thinness of the extraocular muscles in a normal orbit. (Reproduced with permission from the Publisher, Philips Medical Systems Division, Eindhoven, The Netherlands)

Class 5. Corneal involvement. Exophthalmos, lid retraction, and less frequent blinking all contribute to the exposure of the cornea, which can lead to keratitis. Early signs are photophobia, a gritty sensation, blurred vision, and intolerance to contact lenses. The presence of corneal irritation is not by itself a sign of severe ophthalmopathy, because it can often be relieved by the liberal application of eye drops and ointments.

Class 6. Sight loss. Sight loss due to optic nerve damage can be accompanied by visual field defects and impaired color vision.[32] There is no evidence for a direct inflammation of the optic nerve itself, and optic neuropathy is probably due to swelling of the EOM close to the apex of the orbit: 'apical crowding'. The enlarged muscles might very well cause neuropathy by direct pressure on the nerve or its blood supply.[33] This latter possibility is supported by the observation of swelling of the nerve sheath suggesting venous stasis.[16] Another factor is the increase in retrobulbar pressure seen especially in patients with optic neuropathy.[22] This is in agreement with the fact that the presence of optic neuropathy is unrelated to the degree of proptosis.[33] It has often been noticed that the patients with optic nerve involvement have relatively low proptosis readings.[29,34] Koornneef suggested that a well developed, tight orbital septum might preclude proptosis and nature's decompression, resulting in higher retrobulbar pressures and optic neuropathy (Fig. 6).[29]

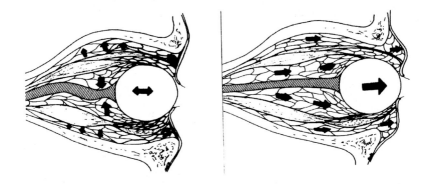

Figure 6. Left, malignant ophthalmopathy, note the tight connective tissue system preventing forward displacement of the globe resulting in a rise in intraorbital pressure (also note the swelling of the muscles at the apex: 'apical crowding'). Right, nonmalignant, proptotic ophthalmopathy. (Reproduced with permission from the Publisher.[29])

The meticulous macroscopic studies by F.F. Rundle and other scientists, together with detailed anatomic investigations have made it possible to at least understand how the clinical signs and symptoms are explained. In the following chapters the present state of the scientific art regarding the other aspects of this disease will be discussed.

4.   REFERENCES

1. Warwick R, Williams PL. Gray's Anatomy. Edinburgh: Longman, 1973; 262-265.

2. Porter JD, Baker RS, Ragusa RJ, Brueckner JK. Extraocular muscles: Basic and clinical aspects of structure and function. Surv Ophthalmol 1995; 39: 451-484.
3. Martinez AJ, Hay S, McNeer KW. Extraocular muscles. Light micorsocopy and ultrastructural features. Acta Neuropath 1976; 34: 237-253.
4. Porter JD, Baker RS. Muscles of a different 'color': The unusual properties of the extraocular muscles may predispose or protect them in neurogenic and myogenic disease. Neurology 1996; 46: 30-37.
5. Sartore S, Mascarello F, Rowlerson A, *et al.* Fibre types in extraocular muscles: a new myosin isoform in the fast fibres. J Musc Res Cell Motility 1987; 8: 161-177.
6. Wieczorek DF, Pariasamy M, Butler-Browne S, Whalen RG, Nadal-Ginard B. Co-expression of multiple myosin heavy chain genes, in addition to a tissue-specific one, in extraocular musculature. J Cell Biol 1985; 101: 618-629.
7. Koornneef L. Orbital espta: anatomy and function. Ophthalmology 1979; 86: 876-880.
8. Koornneef L. Eyelid and orbital fascial attachments and their clinical significance. Eye 1988; 2: 130-134.
9. Rundle FF, Pochin EE. The orbital tissues in thyrotoxicosis: a quantitative analysis relating to exophthalmos. Cli Sci 1944; 5: 51-74.
10. Ettl A, Kramer J, Daxer A, Koornneef L. High resolution Magnetic Resonance Imaging of neurovascular orbital anatomy. Ophthalmology 1997; 104: 869-877.
11. Ringel SP, Wilson B, Barden MT, Kaiser KK. Histochemistry of human extraocular muscle. Arch Ophthalmol 1978; 96: 1067-1072.
12. Schmidt ED, Van der Gaag R, Koornneef L. The retrobulbar immune apparatus. Acta Endocrinol (Copenh) 1989; 121: 17-22.
13. Schmidt ED, Das PK, Van der Gaag R, Tigges AJ, Van der Loos CM, Koornneef L. Potential Antigen-Presenting Cells in normal extraocular muscles demonstrated with double immunoenzyme staining. J Pathol 1991; 164: 135-143.
14. Rundle FF, Finlay-Jones LR, Noad KB. Malignant exophthalmos: a quantitative analysis of the orbital tissues. Australasian Ann Med 1953; 2: 1-8.
15. Feldon SE, Lee CP, Muramatsu K, Weiner JM. Quantitative computed tomography of Graves' ophthalmopathy. Arch Ophthalmol 1985; 103: 213-215.
16. Trokel SL, Jakobiec FA. Correlation of CT scanning and pathologic features of Ophthalmic Graves' disease. Ophthalmology 1981; 88: 553-564.
17. Van der Gaag R, Schmidt ED, Zonneveld FW, Koornneef L. Orbital pathology in thyroid-associated ophthalmopathy. Orbit 1996; 15: 109-117.
18. Forbes G, Gorman CA, Brennan MD, Gehring DG, Ilstrup DM, Earnest IV F. Ophthalmopathy of Graves' disease: Computerized volume measurements of the orbital fat and muscle. AJNR 1986; 7: 651-656.
19. Pappa A, Jackson P, Stone J, *et al.* An ultrastructural and systemic analysis of glycosaminoglycans in thyroid-associated ophthalmopathy. Eye 1998; 12: 237-244.
20. Hufnagel TJ, Hickey WF, Cobbs WH, Jakobiec FA, Iwamoto T, Eagle RC. Immunohistochemical and ultrastrucural studies on the exenterated orbital tissues of a patient with Graves' disease. Ophthalmology 1984; 91: 1411-1419.
21. Kroll AJ, Kuwabara T. Dysthyroid ocular myopathy. Arch Ophthalmol 1966; 76: 244-257.
22. Otto AJ, Koornneef L, Mourits MP, Deen-van Leeuwen L. Retrobulbar pressures measured during surgical decompression of the orbit. Br J Ophthalmol 1996; 80: 1042-1045.
23. Werner SC. Modification of the classification of the eye changes of Graves' disease: recommendations of the ad hoc committee of the American Thyroid Association. J Clin Endocrinol Metab 1977; 44: 203-204.
24. Eden KC, Trotter WR. Lid-retraction in toxic diffuse goitre. Lancet 1942; 2: 386-387.

25. Noh JY, Nakamura Y, Ito K, Inoue Y, Abe Y, Hamada N. Sympathetic overactivity of intraocular muscles evaluated by accomodation in patients with hyperthyroidism. Thyroid 1996; 4: 289-293.

26. Feldon SE, Levin L. Graves' ophthalmopathy: V. Aetiology of upper eyelid retraction in Graves' ophthalmopathy. Br J Ophthalmol 1990; 74: 484-485.

27. Werner SC. The severe eye changes of Graves' disease. JAMA 1961; 177: 81-85.

28. Dobyns BM. Present concepts of the pathologic physiology of exopthalmos. J Clin Endocrinol Metab 1950; 10: 1202-1230.

29. Koornneef L, Schmidt ED, Van der Gaag R. The Orbit: Structure, autoantigens, and pathology. In: Wall J, How J, eds. Graves' ophthalmopathy. Oxford: Blackwell Scientific Publications, 1990: 1-16.

30. Gorman CA. Ophthalmopathy of Graves' disease. N Engl J Med 1983; 308: 453-454.

31. Sergott RC, Glaser JS. Graves' ophthalmopathy. A clinical and immunologic review. Surv Ophthalmol 1981; 26: 1-21.

32. Tanner V, Tregear SJ, Ripley LG, Vickers SF. Automated achromatic contrast and chromatic discrimination sensitivity testing in dysthyroid optic neuropathy. Eye 1995; 9: 352-357.

33. Kennerdell JS, Rosenbaum AE, El-Hoshy H. Apical optic nerve compression of dysthyroid optic neuropathy on computed tomography. Arch Ophthalmol 1981; 99: 807-809.

34. Mourits MP, Koornneef L, Wiersinga WM, Prummel MF, Berghout A, Van der Gaag R. Orbital decompression for Graves' ophthalmopathy by inferomedial, by inferomedial plus lateral, and by coronal approach. Ophthalmology 1990; 97: 636-641.

Chapter 2

Pathogenesis of Graves' ophthalmopathy

Armin E. Heufelder,* Anthony P. Weetman, Marian Ludgate, Rebecca S. Bahn
*Klinikum der Philipps-Universität Marburg, Zentrum für Innere Medizin, Abteilung Innere Medizin mit Schwerpunkt Gastroenterologie, Endokrinologie, Diabetologie; Baklingerstrasse, 35033-Marburg, Germany

1.   INTRODUCTION

Graves' ophthalmopathy (GO) is a medically incurable, chronic autoimmune process that affects the orbital tissues and is tightly linked with autoimmune thyroid diseases, most notably Graves' disease (GD). The close clinical association between immunogenic hyperthyroidism, ophthalmopathy, and pretibial dermopathy suggests that the antigen responsible for these diverse conditions is common to thyroid gland, orbital tissues and pretibial skin.[1,2] Gross examination of orbital tissues in patients with severe, active GO reveals edematous, enlarged extraocular muscle bodies in conjunction with an increased volume of orbital connective and fatty tissue (Chapter 1). Microscopically, two characteristic abnormalities are apparent: the presence of excessive amounts of hydrophilic glycosaminoglycans (GAGs), predominantly hyaluronic acid and chondroitin sulfate, and marked infiltration of the orbital connective tissue and extraocular muscles by immunocompetent cells (macrophages and T lymphocytes, few B cells). The orbital inflammatory process is likely to be driven by T-cells which, in response to an uncertain antigen, access and infiltrate the orbital space via certain adhesion molecules.[1,3] Once recruited, these T cells release numerous cytokines capable of stimulating cell proliferation, GAG synthesis, and generation of new fat cells from orbital adipose precursor cells responding to adipogenic stimuli. Moreover, many of these autocrine and paracrine factors act to alter the expression of an array of immunomodulatory molecules in orbital preadipocyte fibroblasts. During the active, inflammatory stage of the disease, the extraocular muscles are widely separated by proliferating fibroblasts, increased quantities of fibroblast-derived GAG and fluid contained within the expanding perimysial and interstitial connective tissue, whereas the muscle fibers themselves are morphologically intact. Unregulated accumulation of collagen and GAGs as well as the attendant edema are responsible for a rise of the intraorbital pressure, which leads to tissue hypoxia and oxygen free radical damage, followed by intraorbital tissue remodeling.[3] In later stages, fibrosis with restriction and atrophy of the extraocular muscles account for their clinical dysfunction. The varied clinical expressions of GO, including proptosis, extraocular muscle dysfunction, periorbital and lid edema, chemosis and conjunctival congestion, can be explained mechanically by an increase in connective/fatty tissue and extraocular muscle volume within the confines of the bony orbits.

2.   ENVIRONMENTAL AND GENETIC DETERMINANTS

A fundamental step in determining the risk factors for any disease is precise diagnosis. In identifying susceptibility determinants for GO, a major problem is encountered, as there is no clear definition of when a patient has or does not have the condition. Although clinically apparent eye involvement can be found in around 50-60% of patients with Graves' disease (GD), subclinical disease apparent by exophthalmometry, ultrasonography, CT or MR imaging or evaluation of saccadic eye movement fatigue can be seen in at least 90% of cases.[4-7] One is, therefore, left with an unsatisfactory comparison between Graves' patients with obvious GO and those without eye signs or with controls, but few studies have attempted to define precisely their study populations, for instance by imaging. Despite this caveat, there is general agreement that severe GO comprises particularly those features leading to intervention, such as proptosis, diplopia or visual failure, and studies looking at susceptibility determinants in such patients are worthwhile as the results may shed light on our incomplete understanding of pathogenesis.

As with almost all autoimmune diseases, GO is believed to be multifactorial and to depend on the interaction between environmental, genetic and endogenous factors. The latter (anatomical features such as orbital shape, the arrangement of fibrous tissue and other factors) could be important, for instance in unilateral GO, but remain poorly characterized. It also seems highly likely that no single combination of factors will result in GO. Rather, separate combinations may operate in individuals but result in a common presentation. In general one might expect predominant genetic effects to operate mostly during the early part of life, while environmental factors require appropriate exposure to take effect and may therefore exert their influence most strongly in later life.

2.1   Environmental factors

Smoking is the most clearly identified risk factor for GO. Following the impressive observation of increased smoking in a small number of patients,[8] many groups have confirmed that smoking is indeed associated with clinically apparent GO and, to a lesser extent, with GD itself.[9-12] Tobacco consumption is positively associated with the increased risk, and there is an association between the severity of GO and the amount smoked. Moreover, Asians with GD are at lower risk of developing GO than Western Caucasians, itself suggesting a genetic effect from an unidentified locus, but in this population, too, smoking is a risk factor.[13] The reason for the association is unknown. One possibility is that there is a link to the effects of smoking on the thyroid, perhaps through modulation of autoantigen release. Alternatively, smoking causes hypoxia, which increases glycosaminoglycan production by fibroblasts.[14] Finally there may be immunological effects of smoking which are detrimental, particularly through actions on cytokine production, such as IL-1 receptor antagonist.[15] Overall, the relative risk conferred by smoking is around 3. It remains to be established that cessation of smoking is beneficial in respect to GO, although most physicians recommend that this is done.[16]

The type of treatment of the underlying thyroid disease has long been debated as a factor initiating or worsening GO (see Chapter 6). A recent and definitive prospective study[17] has shown that radioiodine is followed by the appearance or worsening of ophthalmopathy more often than after methimazole treatment (15% *vs.* 3%). However, this worsening is usually only transient. Hypothyroidism is one explanation for deterioration of eye signs after treatment, as GO is worse in patients with abnormal thyroid function.[18] However, the specific effects of radioiodine may be more related to radiation effects on T cell populations and other immunological factors, particularly as activated T cells appear in the circulation within weeks after ^{131}I treatment.[19] Several patients have been reported in whom there appeared to be a close temporal relationship between lithium treatment and the development of GO; in one patient there was a dramatic improvement after cessation of lithium.[20] Lithium is known to exacerbate autoimmune thyroid disease and this therefore seems likely to be a real effect, although only of minor significance.

2.2   Genetic factors

Association and linkage studies of genetic susceptibility in GO suffer particularly from the problems of case ascertainment bias, incomplete penetrance and often insufficient power for confidence in the results.

Table 1. Explanation of various terms used in this Chapter

Term	Explanation
Concor- dance Rate	Applied to twin studies, this is an estimate of the frequency of the condition under investigation. A concordance rate below 1 in monozygotic twins must be caused by environmental (non-genetic) factors. The lower the concordance rate, the less important genetic factors are in susceptibility. A concordance rate similar to the population frequency of the condition implies an absence of a genetic contribution. Genetic susceptibility is suggested by a higher concordance rate in monozygotic than dizygotic twins.
Lambda score	The λ statistic is a measure of the risk of a condition developing in a relative of a proband with that condition. Typically siblings are analyzed giving the λs annotation. It is calculated as the frequency of the condition in siblings of a proband, divided by the frequency in the general population. It depends on the prevalence of the condition in the general population as well as in relatives: a strong genetic effect in a common disease will result in a lower λs than the same strength effect in a rarer disease.
Linkage analysis	Used to map disease susceptibility genes. In essence, families with the condition are examined to test whether the disease is associated with any of a series of known markers. In practice, differing alleles at 2 or more loci are examined in various families to see whether these are distributed in a Mendelian fashion, or, instead, are inherited together more frequently, in which case it is most likely that there is linkage. Only a proportion of any set of families is informative, as critical individuals must be doubly heterozygous at the loci to show recombination
Lod score	Abbreviation of logarithm of the odds ratio for linkage, also known as the z score. It is a measure of the strength of linkage between 2 genes and is expressed as the logarithm of the ratio of the 2 likelihoods, L1 and L2. L1 being the probability that the data are the result of 2 loci linked under a specific recombination factor (θ). L2 being the probability that there is no linkage in which case $\theta=0.05$. A Lod score >3 implies linkage.
Pene- trance	Classically, for a penetrant mutant gene, all affected individuals express the phenotype; incomplete penetrance means that it is expressed in some but not all subjects (typically in autoimmune diseases)
Power	Probability of correctly concluding that there is linkage. Used to determine sample size for family and population studies.
Recom- bination Fraction	Recombination takes place when homologous chromosomes cross over at meiosis. The recombination factor θ is a measure of this, with values ranging from 0 (loci so close that they never cross over), to 0.5 (unlimited crossover from distant loci on the same chromosome, or on different chromosomes).

HLA is the most widely studied candidate genetic susceptibility locus in autoimmune disease. Early association studies in Germany and Hungary found an increase in the HLA-B8, DR3 haplotype in Graves' patients with clinically obvious GO, compared to those patients without GO.[21,22] However, studies in Denmark, France and the UK have found no differences, possibly explicable, in the later studies at least, by improvements in the accuracy of typing with molecular methods.[23-26] HLA-DPB1*0201 appears to be a protective allele in both Caucasian and Japanese Graves' patients, as the frequency of this allele is lower in patients with severe GO, but further work is needed to confirm this observation and understand its role.[27,28]

The only other confirmed genetic susceptibility factor in GD is CTLA-4 polymorphism.[29] In a recent study, however, there was no difference in the frequency of the CTLA-4 106bp microsatellite polymorphism, associated with GD overall, in those patients with severe, clinically obvious GO.[30] This association between CTLA-4 gene polymorphism and GD is certainly not unique, extending to autoimmune hypothyroidism, type 1 diabetes and Addison's disease, in a similar fashion to the pervasive association with HLA-DR3. Thus, these two loci may well determine the overall level of autoimmune responsiveness in some way and, at least in the case of HLA-DR3, this seems to extend to effects on the immune function of healthy individuals. Therefore, there is no clear genetic susceptibility factor which is unique to GD, let alone GO, and we will need to understand much more about the genetics of GD itself before we can hope to be really clear about GO.

The magnitude of any underlying genetic effect on disease causation can be judged in several ways. One is the risk ratio to relatives (λ), although this ratio must be used in conjunction with knowledge of population prevalence of disease. Thus, a common disease might be associated with a relatively low relative risk to siblings (λs), but this would still imply an important genetic contribution. A λs of greater than 2 is usually taken as evidence of a genetic effect and the λs for GD is shown in Table 2. The overall impression, notwithstanding the high frequency of GD, is that λs is small; by comparison, λs for rheumatoid arthritis is 8 and for type 1 diabetes is 15. Another measure of the strength of a genetic effect is concordance between monozygotic twins, but this was only 22% in a recent detailed survey.[31] The problems of power and penetrance make it difficult to be confident that this is the best value obtainable, but equally, twins share environmental as well as genetic factors which would tend to inflate the concordance rate.

Against this background, and with two susceptibility loci already detected, it remains to be seen how easily other loci will be detected, particularly by linkage studies with candidate genes or by genome screening. Recent loci linked to GD have been suggested on chromosome 14q31 and Xq21.33-22,[32,33] but the power of these studies has been rather low. For 3 equally contributing genetic loci which are additive rather than multiplicative in their effects, and assuming a (high) λs of 6.0, 140 sib pairs will be needed in a linkage study in GD to have a power of 0.96 with a Lod score of 1.0, whereas 210 pairs will only have a power of 0.81 with a more traditional Lod score of 3.0.

Table 2. Risk ratio for siblings (λs) in GD

| Study | λ sibling | |
	Sister	Brother
Bartels[36]	12.6	2.1
Howel-Evans et al.[37]	5.4	1.2
Stenszky et al.[38]	8.1	not done
Gough (personal communication)	2.5 (combined)	

Since it is very unlikely that the genetic susceptibility in GD will be as simple as 3 additive loci, it can be seen that any approach based on sib pair linkage analysis will need to be huge to have confidence in the results, and that detecting subtle effects in GO will be even more difficult. Nonetheless, the possible detection of an X-linked susceptibility locus[33] is of interest in the context of GO, as there is a clear preponderance of men with severe GO;[34,35] an alternative explanation for this observation may be the higher prevalence of smoking in men.

3.   IMMUNE REACTIONS

Infiltrating immunocompetent cells act to establish and perpetuate the orbital autoimmune process in GO.[3] Immunohistochemical analysis of mononuclear cell infiltrates in orbital tissues of patients with active GO has revealed a predominance of T lymphocytes (CD3[+]) and macrophages, and a smaller percentage of B lymphocytes.[39,40] Both helper/inducer (CD4[+]) and suppressor/cytotoxic (CD8[+]) T lymphocytes are present, with some predominance of the latter. A significant proportion of T-lymphocytes, frequently detected adjacent to blood vessels, are CD3[+]/CD45RO[+] cells, reflecting a subset of memory T-cells and macrophages. Moreover, immunohistochemical characterization of the T cell antigen receptors expressed in situ in GO has revealed that the majority of orbital T cells carry the α/β T cell receptor.[41] Analysis of orbital TcR V region gene repertoires has revealed evidence of limited variability of TcR V gene usage in patients with active GO of recent onset. By contrast, lesser degrees or absence of restriction of TcR V gene usage was found in patients with longstanding, clinically inactive GO, and unrestricted TcR V gene usage was demonstrated in orbital tissue of patients with unrelated orbital conditions, and in peripheral blood lymphocytes of all individuals studied.[41] Of note, comparison of TcR V gene usage between orbital connective/fatty tissue and extraocular muscle did not reveal any major differences, suggesting that the relevant antigenic epitopes may be present in both tissue compartments. Recently, intrathyroidal, orbital and pretibial TcR V gene repertoires have been analyzed in two patients who presented with Graves' disease, severe active GO and PTD.[42] Compared with PBL, marked restriction of TcR V gene usage was detected in thyroid, orbital and pretibial tissue obtained from the first patient, and in orbital and pretibial tissue obtained from the second patient, but not in samples derived from thyroid, orbital and pretibial tissue of two healthy individuals. Despite obvious heterogeneity of the TcR V gene repertoire between these two patients, marked similarities of restricted V gene family usage were noted in T cells present at these distinct sites of either patient. DNA sequencing of dominant TcR Vβ gene families in intra- and extrathyroidal tissues of either patient revealed two major populations of TcRs whose rearrangements shared significant homologies at the amino acid level of junctional regions. Comparison of the CDR3 domains of junctional regions in expanded TcR V gene families revealed several conserved amino acid motifs that were shared by intrathyroidal, orbital and pretibial lymphocytes, but not by peripheral blood lymphocytes. These results indicate that certain populations of intrathyroidal, orbital and pretibial lymphocytes are oligoclonal, and that several clones are present at a high frequency in these distinct sites.[1,3,42] Collectively, these data support the hypothesis that, in GD, common antigenic determinants may drive the immune response against the thyroid gland and certain extrathyroidal sites. While the antigen-driven T-cell response appears to be highly focused during the initiation of the immune response, ongoing tissue destruction and cytokine-induced antigen expression during the later stages of the disease may promote the recruitment of a more diverse spectrum of T cells that use multiple TcR V gene families and react to a variety of tissue-specific and tissue-non-specific antigens.

4. TARGET ANTIGENS AND TARGET CELLS

Efforts to identify relevant orbital autoantigens in GO have suffered from the lack of a valid animal model and from the limited availability of affected human tissue suitable for study. Considerable confusion has been generated by studies that used crude homogenates of non-human orbital tissues. Circulating antibodies against proteins contained in eye muscle (64 kDa) and orbital fibroblasts (23 kDa) are frequently detected in sera of patients with

GO,[43,44] but these antibodies lack both tissue and disease specificity, indicating that they are the products rather than the cause of the orbital inflammatory process. New candidate proteins (63-64 kDa, 1D; 63 kDa, calsequestrin; 67 kDa, flavoprotein; 53 kDa, sarcalumenin; 220 kDa, G2s) have recently been added to this expanding list by J. Wall and collaborators, but it is now clear that antibodies recognizing these proteins are frequently directed against ubiquitous cytoskeletal components that are common to cells outside of the orbits. While this phenomenon may in part reflect the systemic involvement in Graves' disease, these antibodies are likely to arise secondarily as a result of the local inflammatory process, and thus do not qualify as sensitive and specific markers of GO.[1,45,46]

Several studies have addressed the nature of the effector and target cells in the orbits, as well as their interaction within other orbital cell types. T cells obtained from the retrobulbar tissue of patients with GO were shown to specifically recognize, in an MHC class I-restricted manner, autologous orbital fibroblasts, but not crude eye muscle extract, autologous peripheral blood mononuclear cells, allogeneic cells, or purified protein derivative of mycobacterium tuberculosis.[47] These T cells were predominantly of the CD8[+], CD45RO phenotype, revealed little target cell cytotoxic activity, and secreted marked amounts of cytokines upon activation, suggesting that stimulation of fibroblasts, rather than their destruction, may be an important pathogenic mechanism. It was recently demonstrated that proliferation of Graves' intrathyroidal T lymphocytes is strongly stimulated, in a MHC class I-restricted manner, by co-culture with autologous IFNγ-treated Graves' orbital fibroblasts, and to a lesser degree Graves' thyroidal, pretibial myxedema- and Graves' extraocular muscle-derived fibroblasts, but not Graves' abdominal fibroblasts and non-Graves' synovial fibroblasts (Fig.1).

Moreover, recent data suggest that interaction of CD40L on orbital T lymphocytes with CD40 expressed by orbital preadipocyte fibroblasts triggers their release of several important cytokines, chemokines and growth factors (Heufelder *et al.*, manuscript in preparation). Collectively, these data strongly support the notion that, within the orbits, both orbital connective/adipose tissue and stromal cell within extraocular muscle harbor the antigen-bearing cells in GO, and that T cells mainly recognize and stimulate orbital fibroblasts. These cells respond to appropriate stimulation with greater expression of certain immunomodulatory molecules such as MHC class I and class II molecules, intercellular adhesion molecule-1 (ICAM-1) and 72 kDa heat shock protein (HSP72).[48-51] Moreover, similar to their intrathyroidal counterparts, orbital fibroblasts act as potent inhibitors of T cell and B cell apoptosis, thereby extending their encounter with immune effector cells and perpetuating the orbital immune process.[3]

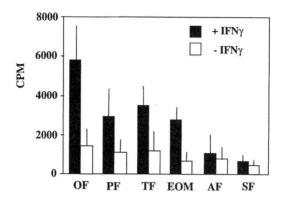

Figure 1. Quantitative analysis of cell proliferation (^{3}H-Thymidin-assay) in Graves' intrathyroidal T lymphocytes during co-culture with autologous fibroblasts obtained from various anatomical locations. Fibroblast monolayers were either untreated or treated with IFNγ (10 U/ml), as indicated. OF=Graves' orbital fibroblasts; PF=pretibial dermopathy-derived fibroblasts; TF=Graves' thyroid fibroblasts; EOM=Graves' extraocular muscle-derived fibroblasts; AF=abdominal fibroblasts; SF= normal synovial fibroblasts (Contributed by A.E. Heufelder).

5.   NEW DATA ON THE TARGET AUTOANTIGEN

In recent years, some progress has been made in clarifying the nature of the target autoantigen in GO. In fact, there is now considerable support for the thyrotropin receptor (TSHR) playing an important role. In many ways, the receptor was always an obvious candidate since GO is most frequently associated with GD and indeed with those patients having highest titers of thyroid stimulating antibodies (TSAb). Patients displaying one or more of these extrathyroidal manifestations frequently develop severe GO, and high concentrations of TSHR stimulating immunoglobulins are usually detected in their sera. Although a close correlation between the presence of TSHR-directed antibodies and the presence or severity of GO has not been established, severe GO frequently occurs in the presence of high concentrations of TSHR-stimulating immunoglobulins.[52] In view of these close links between the thyroidal and extrathyroidal manifestation (GD and GO), if a common antigen is shared between the thyroid gland and the orbital and dermal connective tissue against which the autoimmune attack is directed, the TSHR would appear to be a prime candidate. However, for the TSHR to be implicated it seems reasonable to expect the receptor or a cross reacting protein to be present in the orbit, and also to be able to detect autoreactivity to the receptor in all patients with GO, even in the small number who have no apparent thyroid dysfunction.

The TSHR has long been considered a thyroid-specific protein, and the presence of TSHR in non-thyroid tissues has been controversial. However, a large body of work from several laboratories now suggests that the TSH receptor is expressed in various extrathyroidal sites, including orbital and pretibial tissues.[53-62] The capacity of extrathyroidal TSHR to transmit signals and thereby alter certain metabolic and immunological activities in target cells has been examined by several groups using different assays to demonstrate function. Some studies suggested that TSH and affinity-purified immunoglobulins with high TSHR stimulating activity indeed alter, in a dose-dependent manner, certain metabolic (e.g. adenylate cyclase activity) and immunological functions (e.g. expression of HLA-DR, ICAM-1) in certain non-thyroidal cells such as orbital fibroblasts and transfected, TSHR-positive CHO cells.[63] (Bahn *et al.*, manuscript submitted). Whether or not the extrathyroidal TSHR is capable of transmitting signals must, however, be distinguished from its potential role as an autoantigen, because demonstration that the receptor is functional is not a requirement for it to serve as an autoantigen. Recognition by antigen-specific T cells of multiple epitopes of the TSHR extracellular domain has been demonstrated, but the question of whether or not extrathyroidal TSHR may serve as a target for autoreactive T cells has not been specifically addressed. Future studies designed to examine whether lymphocytes obtained from affected tissues recognize TSHR following processing by local antigen-presenting cells will hopefully resolve this important question. Finally, doubts have been raised as to whether the low levels of TSHR transcripts detected in extrathyroidal tissues may be biologically relevant and sufficient to trigger an immune response.[58,59] However, small quantities of TSHR protein would be sufficient for this purpose, especially as an abundant reservoir of TSHR protein is present within the thyroid gland that allows for the generation of large numbers of antigen-specific T cells. Once the autoimmune process is established, circulating sensitized T cells and antibodies are likely to recognize even small quantities of a similar protein at remote sites.

Many approaches have been applied to demonstrate TSHR transcripts and protein in orbital tissues (see below).[3,64] Several groups of investigators have recently concentrated their efforts on the adipose compartment. Ludgate and colleagues performed Northern blot analysis of orbital fat from a patient with GO.[65] Following extended exposure, the major TSHR transcripts (4.6, 1.7 and 1.3 kb) were clearly visible although the signal from the thyroid was detectable after only 24 hours. Despite loading RNA obtained from the adipose tissue of an entire normal orbit, TSHR transcripts were at the limit of detection. Furthermore, when probed with a house-keeping gene, it was apparent that total RNA content per gram of tissue was more in the GO sample, suggesting that its adipose tissue was more cellular than the normal. Recent studies from T. Smith's group have shown that a subpopulation of orbital fibroblasts, the preadipocyte, is able to differentiate into adipocytes in vitro, although the hormones and/or cytokines responsible have yet to be characterised.[66] Taken together, these data suggests that the GO adipose tissue is more cellular and comprises a higher proportion of preadipocytes differentiating into adipocytes, and that the TSHR is expressed in one of these populations. It is not clear whether the increase in receptor transcripts is restricted to the orbital adipose tissues from GO patients or whether it is present in other patients with hyper- or hypothyroidism.

A logical next step was to determine whether the TSHR transcripts are translated into a protein and expressed at the surface of the cell. Several approaches have been attempted to generate monoclonal antibodies to the TSHR, particularly those recognizing receptor conformation. Genetic immunization has permitted the production of a number of monoclonals[67] and two of them have been applied to cryostat sections of various orbital and other biopsies, in immunocytochemistry. BA8 is specific for the human TSHR but 3G4 also binds to dog and rodent receptors, as evidenced by the dense immunostaining at the basolateral surface of the thyrocyte. Muscle biopsies have been examined from 17 and adipose tissue from 5 patients with GO and compared them with muscle biopsies from 10 strabismus corrections, 1 normal orbital fat and 2 biopsies from patients with pseudotumour. In the GO patients, they observed immunostaining on elongated cells with a fibroblast appearance which were often adjacent to clusters of adipocytes. No such staining was present in the strabismus or pseudotumour samples. In the GO orbital fat specimens only, faint but detectable staining was present in the thin rim of cytoplasm of many of the adipocytes (Ludgate *et al.*, manuscript submitted). The immunoreactivity could be due to a TSHR crossreacting protein although the fact that two different monoclonals gave the same results and coupled with the demonstration of TSHR transcripts in GO orbital fat, implies that it is the receptor protein itself which produces the observed ex vivo immunostaining. The presence of immunoreactivity in two cell populations of differing morphology implies that both preadipocyte and mature adipocyte express the TSHR. As detailed below, preliminary data now suggest that TSHR expressed by orbital preadipocyte fibroblasts is functional in terms of signal transduction (Bahn *et al.*, manuscript submitted).

A frequently cited argument against the TSHR being an important target antigen in GO is the existence of patients having no thyroid dysfunction or testing negative for TSHR autoantibodies, as detected in currently available assays. The paucity of receptor protein has precluded the measurement of antibodies which simply bind to the receptor, as can be done for the other major autoantigens, thyroglobulin and thyroid peroxidase. To further address this issue, Ludgate *et al*. have performed Western blots on the extra-cellular part of the receptor expressed as a fusion protein[68] in bacteria (MBP-ECD), using sera from patients with various autoimmune diseases and in particular 11 GO patients negative for TSAb and thyrotropin binding inhibiting immunoglobulins (TBII). Rather surprisingly, they observed a low level of IgG reactivity to the receptor even in some normal individuals. However, 3/11 GO patients displayed more intense IgG antibody staining than any of the normals to the receptor fusion protein. When detecting IgA antibodies, 6/11 GO patients bound to a degraded fragment of the receptor fusion protein which was also recognized by 3/5 Hashimoto's, only 1/6 GO sera positive for TBII and TSAb, 1/6 sera from Graves' patients without GO and not recognized by sera for 6 patients with systemic lupus erythematosus, 6 patients with multinodular goiter or 12 normal individuals (Ludgate *et al.*, manuscript in preparation). These data can be added to the catalogue of evidence accumulating in favor of the TSHR being expressed outside the thyroid and being implicated not only in TED but also in a rare manifestation of GD, pretibial myxedema (PM), in which elongated fibroblast-like cells in the dermis of PM patients display immunoreactivity with the receptor monoclonals 3G4 and BA8 (Ludgate *et al.*, manuscript submitted). However, if the TSHR is central to GO, it should be possible to induce an animal model of the disease by treating with a receptor preparation or with T cells sensitized to the TSHR.

In recent years, progress has been made in developing animal models of GD. Several approaches have been applied, with varying success in inducing thyroid stimulating antibodies (TSAb), TBII, increased circulating thyroid hormone levels, thyroiditis, and changes in the orbit similar to those seen in GO. Ludgate *et al*. have used three different protocols. Initially the extra-cellular domain (ECD) of the receptor produced in bacteria was used. To aid purification, the ECD was generated fused to the bacterial maltose binding protein (MBP). BALBc mice immunized with MBP-ECD developed thyroiditis and TBII, which was not seen in animals immunized with MBP alone.[1] Genetic immunization, where the cDNA for the full coding region of the human TSH-receptor, in a eucaryotic expression vector is administered intra-muscularly, has also been used. This method results in the in vivo production of receptor on the surface of muscle cells which take up the injected cDNA. Moreover, it results in thyroiditis, TBII, and, in some cases, TSI.[2] Finally, passive transfer has been employed of T cells (splenocytes) sensitized to the receptor in vivo, either by treatment with MBP-ECD, or by genetic immunization followed in each case by priming with MBP-ECD.

The results obtained in these models have generated several important conclusions. First, female mice are more susceptible to disease induction, in agreement with the higher incidence of autoimmunity in women. Second, the type of disease induced varies with the genetic background, particularly the MHC haplotype, with some strains of mice being completely resistant.

Table 3. Thyroiditis and Orbital Pathology in BALBc Recipients of TSH-R primed T Cells (contributed by M. Ludgate)

Thyroiditis + or -	% of infiltrated thyroid interstitium	B:T cell ratio	IL-4 to IFNγ ratio	orbital pathology + or -	% of infiltrated orbital interstitium
Mice examined 8 weeks after transfer of T cells primed with receptor protein (MBP-ECD)					
-	12	0.8	1.32	-	7.6
-	13	0.9	1.43	-	7.3
+	20	1.2	1.98	-	8.8
+	20	1.3	2	-	9.5
+	19	1.3	2.12	-	8.9
+	24	1.7	2.99	+	14.2
+	25	1.8	3.18	+	14.4
+	28	1.8	3.09	+	16.6
+	29	1.9	3.22	+	15.3
+	28	1.9	3.41	+	17.5
Examined 8 weeks after transfer of CD4+ T cells primed with receptor protein (MBP-ECD)					
-	15	0.8	1.33	- 8.7	8.7
+	19	1.2	1.93	- 9.5	9.5
+	20	1.2	1.84	- 8.4	8.4
+	28	1.8	2.53	+ 18	18.0
+	30	1.9	2.61	+ 17.7	17.7
Examined 12 weeks after transfer of T cells primed with receptor protein (MBP-ECD)					
+	26	1.6	3	+	17.2
+	26	1.7	3.26	+	16.6
+	28	1.7	3.41	+	18.6
+	28	1.8	3.42	+	16.4
+	30	1.9	3.5	+	18.7

In BALBc mice, the type of thyroiditis induced is characterized by infiltrating activated T cells and B cells that display immunoreactivity for the cytokines IL-4 and IL-10. In addition, the animals have antibodies to the receptor which are often TBII although the animals have increased levels of circulating total T4. In contrast, in NOD mice the thyroiditis is very destructive with many activated T cells, few B cells and immunoreactivity for IL-2 and IFNγ, the animals having reduced levels of circulating total T4. The BALBc mice develop a Th2 type response and the NOD a Th1 response to the receptor, both resulting in disease. In view of the information obtained from GO patient biopsies indicating the presence of the receptor in the orbit, the investigators went on to examine the orbits of BALBc and NOD mice, both recipients of receptor primed T cells. When compared with the well organized architecture of a normal orbit, no changes were observed in the NOD mice. However, the BALBc orbits appeared totally disorganized, largely the result of edema which disrupted the muscle fibers and contained PAS-positive material. Apart from this, the orbits displayed infiltration by large numbers of mast cells and lymphocytes. These changes were noted in 17/25 BALBc mice and indicate that a Th2 response to the receptor may be required for the development of GO.[72] Orbital pathology did not correlate with levels of circulating total T4 or with TBII levels. To quantitate the thyroiditis and orbital pathology, the surface area occupied by interstitium and ratios of B:T cells and IL-4 : IFNγ were calculated. As can be seen from Table 3, orbital pathology was present only in those BALBc mice with severe Th2 thyroiditis, i.e. with a B:T cell ratio >1.6, IL-4: IFNγ ratio >2.5, and >24% of the surface occupied by interstitium. Severity of thyroiditis increased with time. Does this indicate a temporal requirement, with development of thyroiditis preceding the ocular changes, as occurs in many patients with GO? Since there is evidence that rodent fat in many anatomical locations expresses the TSH receptor, will there be signs of edema or infiltration elsewhere? Clearly, the model requires further characterization, however, it should prove invaluable in dissecting the early processes which occur within the response to the receptor and which results in the development of GO in some but not all GD patients.

6.   ORBITAL ADIPOGENESIS AND TSH RECEPTOR EXPRESSION

An overabundance of adipose tissue both within the contents of the orbits and protruding externally is a prominent feature in many patients with GO.[73-75] Adipocyte precursor cells, called preadipocytes, have been isolated from the stromal-vascular fraction of neonatal and adult human adipose/connective tissues from various regions of the body.[76] These cells are a subpopulation of fibroblasts with the potential to undergo adipocyte differentiation under appropriate tissue culture conditions.[77] It is, therefore, of interest to note that cultures derived from orbital connective tissue contain preadipocytes (comprising 5-10% of the cells) that are capable of responding *in vitro* to adipogenic stimuli.[66] These cells may represent an orbital cell subpopulation that, given appropriate *in vivo* stimuli, can differentiate into mature adipocytes. Adipocyte differentiation of orbital fibroblasts appears to be a restricted phenotypic attribute of these cells, because it was not observed in dermal fibroblasts and perimysial fibroblasts from extraocular muscle. Thus, under appropriate conditions of autocrine and paracrine stimulation, orbital preadipocytes may serve as a pool of precursor cells for orbital tissue volume expansion, and perhaps provide metabolic and immunologic activities of relevance to the evolution of GO.

The autoantigen involved in the hyperthyroidism of GD is known to be the thyrotropin receptor (TSHR). The TSHR is a prime candidate orbital autoantigen because its involvement would help to explain the close clinical and laboratory associations between GO and hyperthyroidism. The concept that adipose cells might express TSHR was first brought forward in 1964 by Rodbell in his demonstration of TSH-stimulated lipolysis in rat epididymal fat cells.[78] In subsequent studies, Kendall-Taylor demonstrated lipolysis in rat fat cells incubated with long acting thyroid stimulator[79] and binding of TSH to porcine orbital connective tissue membranes.[80] Other investigators reported TSH binding to guinea pig adipose and retro-orbital tissues[81] and the presence of TSHR mRNA in guinea pig brown and white adipose tissues.[82] Whether human fat cells express TSHR has been more controversial.[81,83] However, it now appears clear that TSHR is expressed in human neonatal adipocytes, and that this expression declines rapidly with age so as to be undetectable in adult adipocytes.[84]

Recent reports by several laboratories have identified TSHR mRNA, or a variant TSHR transcript, in human GO orbital tissues and cell cultures using the reverse-transcriptase polymerase chain reaction.[53,54,85] Because RNA transcripts detected only by PCR-based amplification of cDNA may have little physiologic relevance, more recent studies have used an RPA (ribonuclease protection assay) for semiquantitative detection of this low abundance mRNA. In these studies, Bahn and colleagues demonstrated the presence of mRNA corresponding to TSHR extracellular domain in uncultured GO orbital adipose/connective tissue specimens, and its absence (or barely detectable presence) in normal orbital fatty connective tissue samples.[86] In further studies, they showed that treatment of cultures with TSH stimulates TSHR expression in late-passage cultures of orbital preadipocyte fibroblasts.[87] These results were interpreted to suggest that a humoral factor present in at least some patients with GD might stimulate TSHR expression in orbital cells (perhaps acting through the TSHR itself). If so, this receptor might be available to act as an orbital autoantigen in GO.

More recent studies have explored the link between adipogenesis and the expression of functional TSHR in orbital preadipocyte fibroblasts. In these studies, confluent late-passage GO and normal preadipocyte fibroblasts were grown to confluence in 6-well plates in medium 199 containing 20% fetal bovine serum (FBS) and antibiotics. Differentiation was carried out using a modification of the protocol reported by Sorisky and colleagues.[66] The differentiation protocol was continued for 8-10 days, during which time the medium was replaced every 3-4 days. Control cultures of orbital fibroblasts were treated in parallel fashion in medium not containing $cPGI_2$, dexamethasone and IBMX, or were maintained in standard medium 199 containing 10% FBS. A significant proportion of mature adipose cells was obtained in the differentiated cultures, while only fibroblast-like cells were apparent in the control cultures. Furthermore, there was a significant increase in cAMP production (96-183 fold) following rhTSH stimulation in the differentiated cultures (Fig. 2). In contrast, there was no significant rhTSH-dependent cAMP production in the undifferentiated cultures. These results suggest that, while cultured orbital preadipocyte fibroblasts do not expresses functional TSHR, these cells have the potential to differentiate into TSHR-bearing cells. Further, it appears that the mature adipocytes within these cultures are the cells expressing this functional receptor.

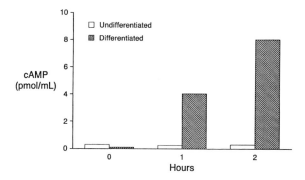

Figure 2. Representative experiment showing cAMP response to rhTSH (1.3×10^{-7} M) stimulation in GO orbital preadipocyte fibroblasts. Late-passage cells from a single GO patient were grown to confluence in medium 199 containing 20% FBS. Cell were then cultured either in defined adipocyte differentiation medium (hashed bars) or in control medium 199 (solid bars) for 8-10 days, during which time the medium was replaced every 3-4 days. The experiment was repeated 4 times using orbital cells from 4 different GO patients with similar results ($p < 0.05$ for differentiated versus undifferentiated cells at both time points). (Contributed by R.S. Bahn).

7. SUMMARY AND PERSPECTIVES

What causes GO is still a mystery, but the disease process results from a complex interplay of genetic and environmental factors. Genes such as those for HLA genes may determine a patient's susceptibility to the disease and the disease severity, but environmental factors, often unknown, may determine its course. Once established, the chronic inflammatory process within the orbital tissues appears to take on a momentum of its own. Given our current state of knowledge, a working scheme for the pathogenesis of GO can be proposed (Fig. 3). On the background of a permissive immunogenetic milieu, circulating T cells in patients with GD, directed against certain antigens on thyroid follicular cells, recognize epitopes of antigens following processing and presentation by dendritic cells and non-professional antigen-presenting cells such as orbital fibroblasts. Of the cell types residing in the orbital tissues, preadipocytes and fibroblasts most likely act as target and effector cells of the orbital immune process.

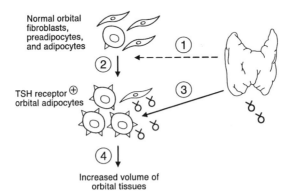

Figure 3. Proposed sequence of events leading to the development of GO. 1) Unknown humoral factors present in the setting of GD circulate to the orbit; 2) Adipogenesis and TSH receptor expression is stimulated within the orbital tissues; 3) TSH receptor-directed T cells infiltrate the orbit and release cytokines that stimulate glycosaminoglycan synthesis and the expression of immunomodulatory proteins by orbital fibroblasts; 4) These changes, along with the increase in orbital adipose tissue, lead to expanded orbital tissue volume and result in the development of clinical disease.

This includes preadipocyte fibroblasts present in the perimysium of extraocular muscles, which do not appear to be immunologically different from those located in the orbital connective tissue. Orbital preadipocyte fibroblasts may be stimulated by unknown circulating or locally produced factors to differentiate into mature adipocytes that express increased levels of TSHR. How autoreactive T cells escape deletion and control by the immune system and come to be directed against a self-antigen presented by cells residing in the thyroid gland and extrathyroidal locations, is currently unknown. Proliferation and expansion of autoreactive T cell clones may be due to molecular mimicry of a host antigen by a microorganism, but this is still speculative. T cell recruitment into the orbital tissues is facilitated by various chemokines and cytokines, which help to attract T cells by stimulating the expression of certain adhesion molecules (e.g. ICAM-1, VCAM-1, CD44) in vascular endothelium and connective tissue cells. These adhesion receptors are known to also play an important co-stimulatory role in activating T cells and facilitating antigen recognition, resulting in amplification of the cellular immune process.[3] Analysis of variable region genes of T cell antigen receptors in orbital T cells of patients with active GO has revealed their restricted TcR V gene usage, suggesting that antigen-driven selection and/or expansion of specific T cells may occur early in the evolution of GO. T cells and macrophages populating the orbital space as well as local fibroblasts and adipocytes are known to synthesize and release a number of cytokines (most likely a Th1-type spectrum) into the surrounding tissue. Cytokines, oxygen free radicals and fibrogenic growth factors, released both from infiltrating inflammatory and residential cells, act upon orbital preadipocytes in a paracrine and autocrine manner to stimulate adipogenesis, fibroblast proliferation, glycosaminoglycan synthesis, and the expression of immunomodulatory molecules. Smoking, a well-known aggravating factor in GO, may enhance tissue hypoxia and exert immunomodulatory effects. The long held hypothesis of a thyroid cross-reactive or shared antigen within the orbital tissues has recently gained significant support by an animal model and by in vitro and ex vivo studies. If confirmed in immunological studies, these results may well explain the localized infiltration of the orbital tissues by autoreactive lymphocytes that share intriguing molecular features with intrathyroidal lymphocytes. The local release of particular cytokines, TSHR-directed antibodies and other factors may further stimulate adipogenesis, glycosaminoglycan synthesis and expression of immunomodulatory proteins within the orbit.[88,89] Other factors, including certain inflammatory cytokines, might act as counterbalancing inhibitors of these effects. However, if the net effect of these changes is to increase the volume of the fatty connective tissues within the orbits, then proptosis, extraocular muscle dysfunction, and periorbital congestion will ensue. Whether this potential sequence of events will finally explain the involvement of the orbit in GD is unknown. Future studies will be aimed at identifying the factors that might modulate adipogenesis in orbital cells and clarifying the link between adipogenesis and TSHR expression in the orbit.

Taken together, a number of important details in the complex pathogenesis of GO have been resolved in recent years, but many challenges remain. Elucidation of the primary antigen and how it is recognized by the immune system will be key issues. Does recognition by T cells of the orbital TSHR indeed initiate the orbital immune response, or does it serve to perpetuate the orbital immune process by binding certain subsets of TSHR autoantibodies and mediating their immunomodulatory effects? What are the important signals that are responsible for attracting T cells to the orbital tissues, and how can they be manipulated therapeutically? Answers to these fundamental questions should soon be forthcoming.

8.   REFERENCES

1. Burch HB, Wartofsky L. Graves' ophthalmopathy: Current concepts regarding pathogenesis and management. Endocr Rev 1993; 14:747-793.
2. Bahn RS, Heufelder AE. Mechanisms of disease: Pathogenesis of Graves' ophthalmopathy. New Engl J Med 1993; 329:1468-1475.
3. Heufelder AE. Retro-orbital autoimmunity. Bailliere's Clin Endocrinol Metab 1997; 11: 499-520.
4. Werner SC, Coleman DJ, Franzen LA. Ultrasonographic evidence of a consistent orbital involvement in GD. New Engl J Med 1974; 308:420-4.
5. Amino N, Yuasa T, Yabu Y, Miyai K. Exophthalmos in autoimmune thyroid disease. J Clin Endocrinol Metab 1980; 51:1232-4.
6. Mauri L, Meienberg O, Roth E, Konig MP. Evaluation of endocrine ophthalmopathy with saccadic eye movements. J Neurol 1984; 231:182-7.
7. Villadolid MC, Yokoyama N, Izumi M, *et al.* Untreated Graves' disease patients without clinical ophthalmopathy demonstrate a high frequency of extraocular muscle (EOM) enlargement by magnetic resonance. J Clin Endocrinol Metab 1995; 80:2830-3.
8. Hägg E, Asplund K. Is endocrine ophthalmopathy related to smoking? Brit Med J 1987; 295:634-5.
9. Bartalena L, Martino C, Marcocci C, *et al.* More on smoking habits and Graves' ophthalmopathy. J Endocrinol Invest 1989; 12:733-7.
10. Shine B, Fells P, Edwards OM, Weetman AP. Association between Graves' ophthalmopathy and smoking. Lancet 1990; 335:1261-3.
11. Tallstedt L, Lundell G, Taube A. Graves' ophthalmopathy and tobacco smoking. Acta Endocrinol 1993; 129:147-50.
12. Prummel MF, Wiersinga WM. Smoking and risk of Graves' disease. JAMA 1993; 269:479-82.
13. Tellez M, Cooper J, Edmonds C. Graves' ophthalmopathy in relation to cigarette smoking and ethnic origin. Clin Endocrinol 1992; 36:291-4.
14. Metcalfe RA, Weetman AP. Stimulation of extraocular muscle fibroblasts by cytokines and hypoxia: possible role in thyroid-associated ophthalmopathy. Clin Endocrinol 1994; 40:67-72.
15. Hofbauer LC, Mühlberg T, König A, Heufelder G, Schworm H-D, Heufelder AE. Soluble interleukin-1 receptor antagonist serum levels in smokers and nonsmokers with Graves' ophthalmopathy undergoing orbital radiotherapy. J Clin Endocrinol Metab 1997; 82:2244-7.
16. Weetman AP, Wiersinga WM. Current management of thyroid-associated ophthalmopathy in Europe. Results of an international survey. Clin Endocrinol 1998; 49:21-8.
17. Bartalena L, Marcocci C, Bogazzi F, *et al.* Relation between therapy for hyperthyroidism and the course of Graves' ophthalmopathy. New Engl J Med 1998; 338:73-8.
18. Prummel MF, Wiersinga WM, Mourits M Ph, Koornneef L, Berghout A, van der Gaag R. Effect of abnormal thyroid function on the severity of Graves' ophthalmopathy. Arch Intern Med 1990; 150:1098-1101.
19. Teng WP, Stark R, Munro AJ, McHardy-Young S, Borysiewicz LK, Weetman AP. Peripheral blood T cell activation after radioiodine treatment for GD. Acta Endocrinol 1990; 122:233-40.
20. Byrne AP, Delaney WJ. Regression of thyrotoxic ophthalmopathy following lithium withdrawal. Can J Psychiatry 1993; 38:635-7.

21. Schleusener H, Schernthaner G, Mayr WR, *et al.* HLA-DR3 and HLA-DR5 associated thyrotoxicosis - two different types of toxic diffuse goiter. J Clin Endocrinol Metab 1983; 56:781-5.
22. Frecker M, Stenszky V, Balazs C, Kozma L, Kraszits E, Farid NR. Genetic factors in Graves' ophthalmopathy. Clin Endocrinol 1986; 25:479-85.
23. Bech K, Lumholz B, Nerup J, *et al.* HLA antigens in GD. Acta Endocrinol 1977; 86:510-15.
24. Allannic H, Fauchet R, Lorcy Y, Gueguen M, LeGuerrier A-M, Genetet B. A prospective study of the relationship between relapse of hyperthyroid GD after antithyroid drugs and HLA haplotype. J Clin Endocrinol Metab 1994; 57:719-22.
25. Kendall-Taylor P, Stephenson A, Stratton A, Papiha SS, Perros P, Roberts DF. Differentiation of autoimmune ophthalmopathy from Graves' hyperthyroidism by analysis of genetic markers. Clin Endocrinol 1988; 28:601-10.
26. Weetman AP, So AK, Warner CA, Foroni L, Fells P, Shine B. Immunogenetics of Graves' ophthalmopathy. Clin Endocrinol 1988; 28:619-28.
27. Weetman AP, Zhang L, Webb S, Shine B. Analysis of HLA-DQB and HLA-DPB alleles in GD by oligonucleotide probing of enzymatically amplified DNA. Clin Endocrinol 1990; 33:65-71.
28. Inoue D, Sato K, Enomoto T, *et al.* Correlation of HLA types and clinical findings in Japanese patients with hyperthyroid Graves' disease: evidence indicating the existence of four subpopulations. Clin Endocrinol 1992; 36:75-82.
29. Yanagawa T, Hidaka Y, Guimaraes V, Soliman M, DeGroot LJ. CTLA-4 gene polymorphism associated with Graves' disease in Caucasian population. J Clin Endocrinol Metab 1995; 80:41-5.
30. Kotsa K, Watson PF, Weetman AP. A CTLA-4 gene polymorphism is associated with both Graves' disease and autoimmune hypothyroidism. Clin Endocrinol 1997; 46:551-4.
31. Brix TH, Christensen K, Holm NV, Harvald B, Hegedüs L. A population-based study of Graves' disease in Danish twins. Clin Endocrinol 1998; 40:397-400.
32. Tomer Y, Barbesino G, Keddache M, Greenberg DA, Davies TF. Mapping of a major susceptibility locus for Graves' disease (GD-1) to chromosome 14q31. J Clin Endocrinol Metab 1997; 82:1645-8.
33. Barbesino G, Tomer Y, Concepcion ES, Davies TF, Greenberg DA. Linkage analysis of candidate genes in autoimmune thyroid disease. II. Selected gender-related genes and the X-chromosome. J Clin Endocrinol Metab 1998; 83:3290-5.
34. Kendler DL, Lippa J, Rootman J. The initial clinical characteristics of Graves' orbitopathy vary with age and sex. Arch Ophthalmol 1993; 111:197-201.
35. Perros P, Crombie AL, Matthews JNS, Kendall-Taylor P. Age and gender influences the severity of thyroid-associated ophthalmopathy: a study of 101 patients attending a combined thyroid-eye clinic. Clin Endocrinol 1993; 38:367-72.
36. Bartels ED. Heredity in Graves' disease. With remarks on heredity in toxic adenoma in the thyroid, non-toxic goitre, and myxoedema. Copenhagen: Einar Munksgaard, 1943: 3-384.
37. Howel-Evans AW, Woodrow JC, McDougall CDM, Chew AR, Evans RW. Antibodies in the families of thyrotoxic patients. Lancet 1967; i:636-641.
38. Stenszky V, Kozma L, Balazs C, Rochlitz S, Bear JC, Farid NR. The genetics of Graves' disease: HLA and disease susceptibility. J Clin Endocrinol Metab 1985; 61:735-40.
39. Heufelder AE, Bahn RS. 1993 Detection and localization of cytokine immunoreactivity in retroocular connective tissue in Graves' ophthalmopathy. Eur J Clin Invest 23: 10-17.
40. Heufelder AE, Bahn RS. Elevated expression in situ of selectin and immunoglobulin superfamily adhesion molecules in retroocular connective tissues from patients with Graves' ophthalmopathy. Clin Exp Immunol 1993; 91: 381-389.

41. Heufelder AE, Herterich S, Ernst G *et al.* Analysis of retroorbital T cell antigen receptor variable region gene usage in patients with Graves' ophthalmopathy. Eur J Endocrinol 1995; 132: 266-277.

42. Heufelder AE, Wenzel BE, Scriba PC. Antigen receptor variable region repertoires expressed by T cells infiltrating thyroid, retroorbital and pretibial tissue in Graves' disease. J Clin Endocrinol Metab 1996; 81: 3733-3739.

43. Bahn RS, Gorman CA, Johnson CM, Smith TJ. Presence of antibodies in the sera of patients with Graves' disease recognizing a 23 kDa fibroblast protein. J Clin Endocrinol Metab 1989; 69: 622-628.

44. Salvi M, Miller A, Wall JR. Human orbital tissue and thyroid membranes express a 64 kDa protein which is recognized by autoantibodies in the serum of patients with thyroid-associated ophthalmopathy. FEBS Letters 1988; 232: 135-139.

45. Kadlubowski M, Irvine MJ, Rowland AC. The lack of specificity of ophthalmic immunoglobulins in Graves' disease. J Clin Endocrinol Metab 1986; 63: 990-995.

46. Kendler DL, Rootman J, Huber GK, Davies TF. A 64 kDa membrane antigen is a recurrent epitope for natural antibodies in patients with Graves' thyroid and ophthalmic abnormalities. Clin Endocrinol 1991; 35: 539-547.

47. Grubeck-Loebenstein B, Trieb K, Sztankay A *et al.* Retrobulbar T cells from patients with Graves' ophthalmopathy are CD8$^+$ and specifically recognize autologous fibroblasts. J Clin Invest 1994; 3: 2738-2743.

48. Heufelder AE, Smith TJ, Gorman CA, Bahn RS. Increased induction of HLA-DR by interferon-gamma in cultured retroocular fibroblasts derived from patients with Graves' ophthalmopathy and pretibial dermopathy. J Clin Endocrinol Metab 1991; 73: 307-313.

49. Heufelder AE, Bahn RS. Modulation of intercellular adhesion molecule-1 (ICAM-1) by cytokines and Graves' IgGs in cultured Graves' retroocular fibroblasts. Eur J Clin Invest 1992; 22: 529-537.

50. Heufelder AE, Wenzel BE, Bahn RS. Cell surface localization of a 72 kilodalton heat shock protein in retroocular fibroblasts from patients with Graves' ophthalmopathy. J Clin Endocrinol Metab 1992; 74: 732-736.

51. Heufelder AE, Wenzel BE, Gorman CA, Bahn RS. Detection, cellular localization and modulation of heat shock proteins in cultured fibroblasts from patients with extrathyroidal manifestations of Graves' disease. J Clin Endocrinol Metab 1991; 73: 739-745.

52. Morris J, Hay ID, Nelson RE, Jiang Nai S. Clinical utility of thyrotropin receptor antibody assays: Comparison of radioreceptor and bioassay methods. Mayo Clin Proc 1988; 63: 707-712.

53. Heufelder AE, Dutton CM, Sarkar G *et al.* Detection of TSH receptor RNA in cultured fibroblasts from patients with Graves' ophthalmopathy and pretibial dermopathy. Thyroid 1993; 3: 297-300.

54. Feliciello A, Porcellini A, Ciullo I *et al.* Expression of thyrotropin-receptor mRNA in healthy and Graves' disease retro-orbital tissue. Lancet 1993; 342: 337-338.

55. Endo T, Ohno M, Kotani S *et al.* Thyrotropin receptor in non-thyroid tissues. Biochem Biophys Res Com 1993; 190: 774-779.

56. Hiromatsu Y, Sato M, Inoue Y *et al.* Localization and clinical significance of thyrotropin receptor mRNA expression in orbital fat and eye muscle tissues from patients with thyroid-associated ophthalmopathy. Thyroid 1997; 6: 553-562.

57. Heufelder AE Involvement of the orbital fibroblast and TSH receptor in the pathogenesis of Graves' ophthalmopathy. Thyroid 1995; 5: 331-340.

58. Paschke R, Elise R, Vassart G, Ludgate M. Lack of evidence supporting the presence of mRNA for the thyrotropin receptor in extraocular muscle. J Endocrinol Invest 1993; 16: 329-332.

59. Paschke R, Metcalfe A, Alcalde L *et al*. Presence of nonfunctional thyrotropin receptor variant transcripts in retroocular and other tissues. J Clin Endocrinol Metabol 1994; 79: 1232-1233.

60. Perros P & Kendall-Taylor P. Demonstration of thyrotropin-binding sites in orbital connective tissue: possible role in the pathogenesis of thyroid-associated ophthalmopathy. J Endocrinol Invest 1994; 17: 163-170.

61. Spitzweg C, Joba W, Hunt N, Heufelder AE. Analysis of human thyrotropin receptor gene expression and immunoreactivity in human orbital tissue. Eur J Endocrinol 1997; 136: 599-607.

62. Stadlmayr W, Spitzweg C, Bichlmair AM, Heufelder AE. Full length TSH receptor transcripts and TSH receptor-like immunoreactivity in orbital and pretibial fibroblasts of patients with Graves' ophthalmopathy and pretibial dermopathy. Thyroid 1997; 7:3-12.

63. Heufelder AE, Bahn RS. Evidence for the presence of a functional TSH receptor in retroocular fibroblasts from patients with Graves' ophthalmopathy. Exp Clin Endocrinol 1992; 100:62-67.

64. Paschke R, Vassart G, Ludgate M. Current evidence for and against the TSH receptor being the common antigen in Graves-disease and thyroid-associated ophthalmopathy. Clin Endocrinol 1995; 42:565-9.

65. Crisp MS, Lane C, Halliwell M, WynfordThomas D, Ludgate M. Thyrotropin receptor transcripts in human adipose tissue. J Clin Endocrinol Metab 1997; 82:2003-5.

66. Sorisky A, Pardasani D, Gagnon A, Smith TJ. Evidence of adipocyte differentiation in human orbital fibroblasts in primary culture. J Clin Endocrinol Metab 1996; 81:3428-31.

67. Costagliola S, Rodien P, Many M-C, Ludgate M, Vassart G. Genetic immunization against the human thyrotropin receptor causes thyroiditis and allows production of monoclonal antibodies recognizing the native receptor. J Immunol 1998; 160:1458-65.

68. Costagliola S, Alcalde L, Ruf J, Vassart G, Ludgate M Overexpression of the extracellular domain of the thyrotropin receptor in bacteria - production of thyrotropin-binding inhibiting immunoglobulins. J Mol Endo 1994; 13:11-21.

69. Costagliola S, Many M-C, Stalmans-Falys M, Tonacchera M, Vassart G, Ludgate M. Recombinant TSHR and the induction of autoimmune disease in BALBc mice, a new animal model. Endocrinology 1994; 135:2150-2159.

70. Costagliola S, Many M-C, Stalmans-Falys M, Vassart G, Ludgate M. The autoimmune response induced by immunizing female mice with the human TSHR varies with the genetic background. Mol Cell Endocrinol 1995; 115:119-206.

71. Costagliola S, Many M-C, StalmansFalys M, Vassart G, Ludgate M. Transfer of thyroiditis, with syngeneic spleen-cells sensitized with the human thyrotropin receptor, to naive balb/c and nod mice. Endocrinology 1996; 137:4637-4643.

72. Many M-C, Costagliola S, Detrait M, Denef J-F, Vassart G, Ludgate M. Development of an animal model of autoimmune thyroid eye disease. J Immunol 1999; 162:4966-4974.

73. Peyster RG, Ginsberg F, Silber JH, Adler LP. Exophthalmos caused by excessive fat: CT volumetric analysis and differential diagnosis. AJNR 1986; 7:35-40.

74. Forbes G, Gorman CA, Brennan MD, Gehring DG, Ilstrup DM, Earnest F. Ophthalmopathy of GD: computerized volume measurements of the orbital fat and muscle. AJNR 1986; 7:651-656.

75. Hufnagel TJ, Hickey WJ, Cobbs WH, Jacobiec FA, Iwamoto T, Eagle RC. Immunohistochemical and ultrastructural studies on the exenterated orbital tissues of a patient with GD. Ophthalmology 1987; 91:1411-1419.

76. Chen X, Hausman DB, Dean RG, Hausman GJ. Differentiation-dependent expression of obese (ob) gene by preadipocytes and adipocytes in primary cultures of porcine stromal-vascular cells. Biochim Biophys Acta 1997; 1359:136-142.

77. Wiederer O, Löffler. Hormonal regulation of the differentiation of rat adipocyte precursor cells in primary culture. J Lipid Res 1987; 28:649-658.
78. Rodbell M. Metabolism of isolated fat cells. I. Effects of hormones on glucose metabolism and lipolysis. J Biol Chem 1964; 239:375-380.
79. Kendall-Taylor P, Munro DS. The lipolytic activity of long-acting thyroid stimulator. Biochim Biophys Acta 1971; 231:314-319.
80. Perros P, Kendall-Taylor P. Demonstration of thyrotropin binding sites in orbital connective tissue: Possible role in the pathogenesis of thyroid-associated ophthalmopathy. J Endocrinol Invest 1994; 17:163-170.
81. Davies TF, Teng CS, McLachlan SM, Smith BR, Hall R. Thyrotropin receptors in adipose tissue, retro-orbital tissue and lymphocytes. Mol Cell Endocrinol 1978; 9:303-310.
82. Roselli-Rehfuss L, Robbins LS, Cone RD. Thyrotropin receptor messenger ribonucleic acid is expressed in most brown and white adipose tissues in the guinea pig. Endocrinology 1992; 130:1857-1861.
83. Mullin BR, Lee G, Ledley FD, Winand RJ, Kohn LD. Thyrotropin interactions with human fat cell membrane preparations and the finding of a soluble thyrotropin binding component. Biochem Biophys Res Commun 1976; 69:55-62.
84. Marcus C, Ehren H, Bolme P, Arner P. Regulation of lipolysis during the neonatal period: Importance of thyrotropin. J Clin Invest 1988; 82:1793-1797.
85. Mengistu M, Lukes YG, Nagy EV *et al.* TSH receptor expression in retroocular fibroblasts. J Endocrinol Invest 1994; 17:437-441.
86. Bahn RS, Dutton CM, Natt N, Joba W, Spitzweg C, Heufelder AE. Thyrotropin receptor expression in Graves' orbital adipose/connective tissues: Potential autoantigen in Graves' ophthalmopathy. J Clin Endocrinol Metab 1998; 83:998-1002.
87. Bahn RS, Dutton CM, Joba W, Heufelder AE. Thyrotropin receptor expression in cultured Graves' orbital preadipocyte fibroblasts is stimulated by thyrotropin. Thyroid 1998; 8:193-196.
88. Smith TJ, Wang HS, Evans CH. Leukoregulin is a potent inducer of hyaluronan synthesis in cultured human orbital fibroblasts. Am J Physiol 1995; 268:C382-C388.
89. Smith TJ, Ahmed A, Hogg MG, Higgins PJ. Interferon-gamma is an inducer of plasminogen activator inhibitor type 1 in human orbital fibroblasts. Am J Physiol 1992; 263:C24-C29.

Chapter 3

Assessment of disease severity

James A. Garrity,* Caroline B. Terwee, Steven E. Feldon, Wilmar M. Wiersinga
*Department of Ophthalmology, Mayo Clinic, Rochester, MN, USA

1. INTRODUCTION

Assessing the severity of Graves' ophthalmopathy is deceivingly difficult. Some of the initial attempts to assess disease severity were based on the NO SPECS (Table 1; Chapter 1).[1] While the idea of a simple numerical index to classify and compare disease severity is appealing, one must recall that this score is a composite of several different observations and measurements. It is exactly for this reason that a composite index should not be used for assessments and reporting results since different parameters can change, in either direction, with no net change in the index score. The optimal method of disease assessment is dependent upon the intent of the measurement. For example, with an individual patient, progression or regression of symptoms and signs of disease is most critical for determining effectiveness. For clinical studies, the amount and location of soft tissue involvement or the "amount" of diplopia may be most relevant for categorizing patients. For patients, being able to function at home or on the job are the most important aspects. The conflict in assessing severity is epitomized by the patients whose CT scans are shown in Figures 1 and 2. One patient has enlargement of all extraocular muscles, but no diplopia while the other patient has intractable diplopia with less enlarged muscles. Furthermore, given that the natural history of the disease consists of a variable period of progressing symptoms and signs over several months followed by a period of stability or improvement, how can the role of immunomodulatory therapy and the optimal time for surgical rehabilitation (e.g. strabismus surgery) be established? (Figs. 1,2; Chapter 4) Depending on the issue, severity of disease can be described utilizing several different techniques. The purpose of this chapter is to characterize the various techniques available and to identify the appropriateness of each for the question at hand.

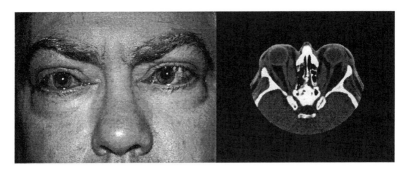

Figure 1. A patient with congestive ophthalmopathy but no diplopia and the corresponding axial CT scan showing enlargement of the medial and lateral rectus muscles. Reproduced with permission from the patient. (Contributed by J.A. Garrity)

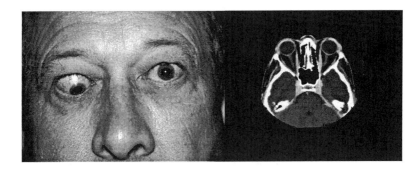

Figure 2. Patient with white, quiet appearing eyes and continuous diplopia and the corresponding axial CT scan showing much less muscle enlargement than in Figure 1 (there was correspondingly similar involvement of the vertical muscles in each patient and CT scan). Reproduced with permission from the patient. (Contributed by J.A. Garrity)

1.1   Assessment of Disease Activity

We define disease activity as the *ongoing* pathological or immunological changes occurring in orbital tissues. Such changes may occur with or without alteration of a patient's clinical symptoms or signs. Usually, an immunologically mediated process is implicated in disease activity; however, there is accumulating evidence that passive venous congestion may also play a substantive role. By definition, a single examination to determine clinical symptoms and signs probably cannot be utilized to assess activity of disease, however, one may infer activity on the basis of a changing examination. Tests of disease activity are provided primarily by imaging techniques, but there is also interest in biochemical markers of disease activity. Serum levels of thyroid stimulating immunoglobulins, when assayed by a bioassay instead of a radioreceptor assay do show a correlation with severity of disease.[2] Glycosaminoglycans can be measured in both the plasma and the urine,[3-6] and were found to be increased in Graves' ophthalmopathy patients compared to controls. These and other parameters are extensively discussed in Chapter 4.

Standardized ultrasound A-scans can be used to assess certain tissue characteristics based upon reflected acoustic waves. Reflectivity in the extraocular muscles changes as a function of tissue edema and cellular infiltration.[7] For example, Prummel *et al.*[8] showed that a low reflectivity on standardized A-scan may be a valid means of assessing activity of disease. Ultrasonographic examinations are best done by operators experienced in the performance and interpretation of the study. The relative rarity of experienced ultrasonographers also limit the utility of this method. MRI offers the potential of being able to estimate disease activity although cost and availability are current limitations of this modality. Pulse sequences that examine T_2 relaxation times can estimate the water content of tissues. When examining the extraocular muscles, normal T_2 relaxation times might imply burned out, fibrotic disease with normal or low water content, whereas prolonged T_2 relaxation times might suggest ongoing inflammation with tissue edema possibly amenable to immunosuppression or radiation therapy. Using a .28 Tesla magnet, some reports noted a correlation between the T_2 relaxation time and a response to immunosuppressive treatment.[9,10] Short tau inversion recovery (STIR) is another MRI pulse sequence which can be used to estimate water content of tissues. Comparing the EOM signal to control tissues, two studies found that a high signal intensity ratio was associated with disease activity.[11,12] The last imaging study to be considered is octreotide scintigraphy, which may visualize active eye disaese.[13-16]

It is easy to become enthusiastic over imaging studies although one should not overlook the clinical examination. Mourits *et al.*[18] developed a Clinical Activity Score (CAS),[17] which could predict the therapeutic outcome with 86% specificity, 55% sensitivity, 80% positive predictive value and a negative predictive value of 64%. One must interject a few words of caution regarding over interpretation of clinical signs, however. Redness and chemosis, which can be associated with active inflammation, are also features of passive orbital congestion. We and others have observed massive chemosis virtually resolve within a few days following orbital decompression which implies more passive congestion rather than active inflammation. Likewise, progressive diplopia, which is an indication of asymmetric extraocular muscle involvement between the eyes, has been associated with active disease. Fibrosis of the extraocular muscles, which can be considered a healing response, can also affect the extraocular muscles asymmetrically and give rise to symptomatic diplopia. Pain, without being further characterized, could be considered superficial and due to corneal exposure from non-active disease related lid causes or could be a deeper aching type of discomfort. The deeper type of pain may be seen in active ophthalmopathy or in states associated with passive orbital congestion not related to active disease itself.

2.   HOW TO ASSESS DISEASE SEVERITY

The concept of disease severity is relative rather than absolute. This is also a function of the question being asked such as cosmetic or functional and who is asking the question such as the clinician or the patient. The presence of an optic neuropathy may be an exception, however. There is general agreement that all cases of optic neuropathy are representative of "severe" disease. There are many parameters by which one can base a determination of severity. Feldon *et al.*[19-21] examined clinical signs and compared these to extraocular muscle volumes determined by CT scanning. Of the parameters scrutinized, (proptosis, periorbital swelling, lid retraction, lid lag, ocular ductions, and optic nerve function), total muscle volume on CT scan and limitation of ocular ductions were found to have an association with subsequent development of optic neuropathy.[22]

Indeed much of what clinicians and patients associate with disease severity is a manifestation or derivative of extraocular muscle involvement. Swelling of the retrobulbar muscles and connective tissues can be considered "primary events".[23] Other manifestations such as proptosis, periorbital swelling, lid retraction, lid lag, diplopia and even optic neuropathy are derivatives of the initial swelling. Since assessment of severity is a relative rather than an absolute concept, there probably are no direct measures of severity but rather one must use indirect means. When considering the assessment of extraocular muscle involvement, there are at least three methods by which one can measure, by clinical testing, by ultrasound, radiographically.

2.1   Clinical assessment of diplopia

Clinically, there are several tests available to assess and follow the Graves' patient with diplopia. The tests can provide an overview of "severity" and one can infer "activity" on the basis of changing examinations. One of these tests is the Hess screen or a Lancaster Red-Green screen. In a Lancaster Red-Green evaluation, a red lens is placed before the right eye and a green lens is placed before the left eye. The examiner then points a red light projector in various positions of gaze and the patient tries to superimpose their green light projector on top of the examiners light. Results with the right eye as the fixating eye are read off the screen directly. The patient and the examiner then switch lights and the measurements are repeated except now the left eye is the fixating eye. These tests provide an objective description of the diplopia in various positions of gaze and can be serially compared.

Table 1. Quantitative measurements for clinical assessment of disease severity

Item	Method
Lid aperture, lagophthalmos	In mm by a ruler
Proptosis	In mm by a Hertel exophthalmometer, or by CT scan
Diplopia	Hess or Lancester Red-Green screen, field of single binocular vision
Extraocular muscle motility	Goldmann or modified hand perimeter
	Range of motion in various directions of gaze
Optic nerve function	Visual acuity
	Visual field defects
	Color vision
	Pupillary function

A diplopia field is a more representative test of the patient's functional ability. In this test the field of single binocular vision can be plotted on a Goldmann perimeter. The head is centered within the bowl of the perimeter and the test light is moved from the center of vision to the periphery. The patient follows the test light and reports as soon as it becomes double. A normal diplopia field is shown in figure 3. This is also the test used to determine ocular disability in terms of extraocular motility. The test is more correctly a measure of symmetry, as very severe, but symmetric disease may produce normal appearing results. Diplopia fields can also be scored, with different scores assigned to each part of the visual field, and followed.[24] Fells et al.[25] state that Hess screen results and fields of single binocular vision (diplopia fields) are their most useful tools to assess and follow their diplopia patients. Recording of subjective diplopia results should make reference to primary gaze and the reading position since these are the two most important positions of gaze. One might use the following algorithm:

An algorithm for reporting diplopia results emphasizing primary gaze and the reading position.

A. None
B. Diplopia when tired or when first awakening
C. Diplopia at extremes of gaze
D. Continuous diplopia correctable with prisms
E. Continuous diplopia not correctable with prisms

Monocular ductions can also be measured and in fact these measurements might give a better idea of the disease status in terms of extraocular muscle involvement.[23] From a practical standpoint however, the measurement efforts have been difficult which partially explains why this examination is not used in everyday practice.[25] Feldon *et al.* used a ruler to measure extraocular excursion.[20] Mourits *et al.* measured ductions with a modified hand perimeter and watching for the light reflex to move from the center of the pupil as the endpoint.[26] Gerling *et al.* used a Goldmann perimeter with a I/4e target and then watched for the endpoint of pursuit movement as the endpoint for measurement determinations.[27]

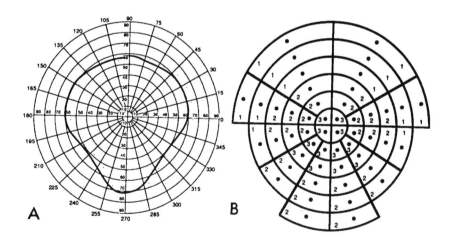

Figure 3. Normal diplopia field (A) with scoring template (B). Note that central values and downgaze are weighted more heavily. (Reproduced with permission from the Publisher.[24])

All of the above methods just measured ductions in 4 directions (abduction, adduction, elevation and depression). It is the feeling of one of the authors (JAG) and others[28] that upgaze and downgaze are not truly representative measurements since up and downgaze are hybrid movements. Downgaze is a mixture of inferior rectus and superior oblique function whereas upgaze is a mixture of superior rectus and inferior oblique activity. We would propose that monocular ductions be measured in 6 cardinal positions of gaze on the perimeter (0°, 45°, 135°, 180°, 225°, and 315°). With the eye slightly abducted, superior and inferior rectus function alone is measured and with the eye slightly adducted, one can assess isolated oblique activity. Unpublished data from the Mayo group was very reproducible in terms of inter and intra observer determinations. The Mayo group used a Goldmann perimeter and determined a target size for each patient to give a 20-degree isopter to emphasize macular fixation. This target was then moved out along the 6 cardinal axes until the patient lost sight of it at which point the measurement was made. The method of Gerling and associates is probably easier to perform.

2.2 Imaging techniques

Ultrasound examinations use a standardized A-mode method to measure maximum diameter of extraocular muscles. The probe is directed toward the widest portion of the muscle. The width of the echographic envelope can be measured directly. In the hands of an experienced orbital ultrasonographer (a relative rarity), the test is relatively reliable, accessible, and inexpensive. On the other hand, numerous authors have reported a wide range of values representing normal values for the different rectus muscles (Table 2). Furthermore, Demer and Kerman[29] compared high resolution MRI with surface coils to standardized echography in the determination of maximum transverse extraocular muscle diameters. The correlation between transverse muscle diameters as measured by echography and that measured by MRI was low. The source of this discrepancy is uncertain, since both techniques are subject to imaging artifacts. In the high-resolution MR images, the muscles had a tear drop shape, perhaps the widest part of the extraocular muscle is not consistently imaged with the ultrasound technique. A possible measure of disease severity over time could be determined by serial measurements of one rectus muscle, using ultrasound, CT or MRI techniques. There is some risk in following only one muscle and making generalized assumptions about overall disease severity. Feldon and Weiner[19] demonstrated a highly significant increase in medial and lateral rectus volumes (P<0.005) and severity (class) of clinical disease. They also showed that volume of the medial rectus muscle did correlate with total muscle volume. In some recent unpublished data from the Mayo orbital radiation therapy study, the maximum transverse diameters of the lateral and medial rectus muscles separately were plotted against the total muscle volume. The coefficient of correlation for medial rectus data was only 0.47 and the coefficient of correlation for lateral rectus data was 0.29. Thus, disease in one muscle may not predict disease in other muscles, leading to a false impression regarding changes in disease severity. Assessment of the total muscle volume is preferred for making accurate volume statements.

Table 2. Reported variance in mm for normal extraocular muscles

Author, ref	Medial	Lateral	Superior	Inferior
McNutt, 77	5.20	5.12	4.58	4.45
Ossoinig, 78	5.4	5.3	5.4	4.3
Willinsky, 79	<3.6	<3.6	-	-
Given-Wilson, 80	4.07	-	-	-
Frazier-Byrne, 81	4.7	3.8	6.7	3.6
Demer, 29	6.08	5.18	6.05	4.71

3.   ASSESSMENT OF DISEASE SEVERITY FROM THE PERSPECTIVE OF THE PATIENT.

From the patients' perspective, clinical measures like muscle volume or monocular ductions are of limited interest; they often correlate poorly with physical, emotional and social functioning in daily life.[30] Recently, this was demonstrated in patients with Graves' ophthalmopathy. Gerding *et al.*[31] found low correlation between the severity or activity of Graves' ophthalmopathy and physical, emotional and social functioning, as measured with a general quality of life questionnaire, the MOS-24 described by Stewart.[32] The low correlation between objective clinical measures and the subjective experience of the patient can be explained by a model of patient outcomes, introduced by Wilson and Cleary.[33] (Fig. 4) Measures of disease status can be thought of as existing on a continuum of different levels of outcome with increasing complexity. Clinical (biological or physiological) measures are on the left side of the model. The perception of these clinical findings by the patient are expressed in perceived symptoms, which can lead to functional limitations in daily activities, which influences the experienced health (general health perceptions) and overall quality of life. The different levels of outcome are causally related but are influenced by personal factors such as previous experiences, expectations, coping strategies, and characteristics of the environment such as social relationships and the physician-patient relationship. The more one moves to the right of the model, the larger the influence of personal and environmental factors and the correlation with clinical measures becomes weaker. This model explains why two people with the same clinical disease status can have a very different perception of their health and quality of life.

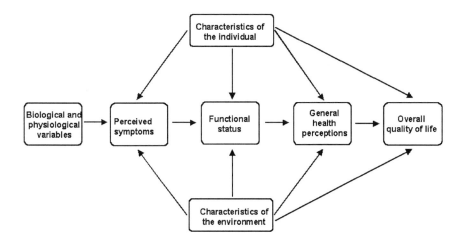

Figure 4. A model of patient outcomes, adapted from Wilson and Clearly[33]

3.1 Do physicians need to worry about quality of life?

In general, delaying or preventing mortality or morbidity is considered sufficient reason to administer a treatment (provided there is a reasonably quality of the extended life). However, when the goal of treatment is to improve functioning and to make patients feel better (rather than to prolong life), clinical measures are often surrogate outcomes for what we really want to measure, the effect of treatment on patients' lives.[34] Since 1948, when the World Health Organization defined health as being not only the absence of disease and infirmity but also the presence of physical, mental, and social well-being, clinicians have come to recognize the importance of direct measurement of how patients are feeling and how they are able to function in daily life.[34,35] Because clinicians are most interested in those aspects of quality of life that are directly related to health (excluding non-medical issues like finances, environmental factors etc.), they refer to health-related quality of life (HRQL), which restricts the focus to perceived symptoms, functional status and general health perceptions in the model of patient outcomes.[33,34]

In 1992, a joint committee of the European, Latin-American, American, Japanese and the Asia-Oceania Thyroid Associations recommended the inclusion of self-assessment of the eye condition by the patient in the evaluation of treatment effects.[36] Now, seven years later, a review of the literature yielded the following efforts.

Already in 1989 Prummel *et al.*[37] introduced the Subjective Eye Score as a secondary outcome measure in clinical trials, by asking patients to rate their eye condition on a scale from 1 to 10 before and after treatment. Although never validated, this rating scale has been used in several studies thereafter.[37-40] Comparable rating scales have been used in later studies. In a small study of 13 patients who underwent decompression, patients were asked to rate their discomfort before and after surgery on a Visual Analog Scale (which is usually a 10 cm line), stretching from "none" to "severe".[41] A comparable linear scale from 0 to 100 was used by Seegenschmiedt *et al.*[42] to measure the subjective degree of improvement in 60 patients after radiotherapy.

Kung and coworkers[43] included subjective assessment of appearance, eye discomfort, diplopia, and visual acuity on a scale of best, improvement, no change, or worse in their study on somatostatin versus corticosteroid in 18 patients. In another small study on 8 patients receiving intravenous methylprednisolone pulse therapy, patient self-assessment of the same aspects was recorded, but it was not reported how this was measured.[44] Recently, an Italian group was the first to include patient's assessment (defined as the degree of interference with daily activities) as a minor criterion in their primary outcome measure of treatment success. However, it was not reported how this was measured and no data on patient's assessment were given in the paper.[45]

Several groups have used some kind of follow-up questionnaire to measure patient satisfaction with treatment results. A Mayo Clinic study evaluated 491 patients who underwent orbital decompression by questionnaire including questions about eye comfort, satisfaction with the appearance of the eyes and overall satisfaction with status of the eyes at a median of 12 years postoperatively.[46-49] A comparable questionnaire was used to describe the long-term follow up of an incidence cohort of 120 patients with newly diagnosed Graves' ophthalmopathy.[50] Other investigators have used questionnaires or telephone interviews to measure treatment satisfaction.[51-55] During the past few years, a group from the Academic Medical Center in Amsterdam performed several studies on quality of life in patients with GO, which will be discussed in greater detail below.[31,56,57]

In summary, two kind of approaches are seen: some authors use rating scales to measure patients' assessment of their eye condition, while others focus on patient satisfaction with treatment results. Although treatment satisfaction is often used as a measure of quality of life and can be an important determinant of quality of life, it might often be more an indication of the willingness to please the doctor. Also, it does not measure (changes in) the amount of discomfort or functional impairments and therefore offers little indications for future direction of treatment. Also, it has been shown that retrospective measurement of satisfaction with care is more influenced by the present health status than by the extent of improvement by treatment.[58] Rating scales may be better instruments for patient assessment of their disease, but only if used outside the physician-patient relationship to avoid willingness to please the doctor.

Either rating scales or other kind of self-assessment questionnaires can be used to assess an overall valuation of the eye condition (as in the Subjective Eye Score) or to value different aspects of the disease separately, such as diplopia and appearance, depending on the research question. Because HRQL is considered a multi-dimensional concept comprising physical, emotional and social aspects, most researchers measure each aspect separately.[34,35,59,60] However, when focussing on separate aspects of disease, it should be secured that all relevant aspects that can be affected, either positively or negatively, are being measured to obtain a correct profile of the HRQL.[34,35] Also, referring to the model of patient outcomes, the outcome level of interest should be decided and reported, which can be either perceived symptoms (e.g. pain, diplopia), or the consequences of these symptoms on functional abilities (e.g. carrying out daily activities) or on general perceived health (overall rating). When assessing change (for example due to treatment), it is advised to measure HRQL before and after treatment, instead of a direct estimation of change. It has been shown that patients don't really remember their initial state and as a consequence tend to overestimate their treatment effect.[61] Finally, reliability and validity of the used instruments should be assessed.[34] In most of the above mentioned studies, patient assessment was performed on an ad hoc basis, without considering the outcome level of interest, the relevant dimensions to be measured, and none of the instruments used was ever validated as a measure of HRQL.

In other disease areas, short, simple, self-assessment questionnaires to be filled in by the patients themselves, are widely used to measure HRQL. Several internationally used validated questionnaires are available. A distinction should be made between general and disease-specific questionnaires.[62] General HRQL questionnaires are mostly multi-dimensional and designed to measure the most important aspects of HRQL that apply to many different impairments patients and populations. Some of these questionnaires are translated into many languages. Examples are the

Medical Outcomes Study short-form measures (SF36 or MOS-24),[32,63,64] the
Sickness Impact Profile (SIP),[65] and the Nothingham Health Profile (NHP).[66]

General HRQL questionnaires are useful to compare different patient
populations. In a descriptive study of Gerding and coworkers[31], the MOS-24
was filled in by 70 patients who visited the combined outpatient clinic of the
Orbital Center and the Department of Endocrinology for the first time.
Twenty-four questions were completed regarding seven different aspects of
HRQL, all scored from 0 to 100, higher scores indicating better health.
Graves' ophthalmopathy patients were compared with patients with other
chronic conditions (diabetes, inflammatory bowel disease (IBD),
emphysema, and heart failure) and with a comparison population of patients
without any chronic conditions (Table 3). Graves' ophthalmopathy patients
showed a markedly decreased HRQL compared with the comparison group
of patients without any chronic conditions. Scores were 6 to 28 points (8%-
36%) lower on all aspects of HRQL. HRQL scores were comparable with
those of patients with IBD, but lower than those of patients with diabetes,
emphysema, or even heart failure. These results show that Graves'
ophthalmopathy has a major impact on daily functioning and well being,
especially on physical functioning and general health perceptions. Mental
health was surprisingly less affected.

Table 3. Mean (SD) MOS-24 scores in patients with Graves' ophthalmopathy (GO), in Dutch
patients with inflammatory bowel disease (IBD; De Boer *et al.*[83]), in patients with other
chronic conditions, as well as in a comparison population (controls) without chronic
conditions. *Stewart *et al.*[82] Bodily pain scores were transformed (higher score=less pain).
NA, not available.

Health measure	GO N=70	Controls* N=2,595	IBD N=268	Diabetes* N=844	Emphyse ma* N=731	Heart failure* N=297
Physical functioning	58 (31)	86	73 (28)	78	73	64
Role functioning	72 (40)	87	61 (43)	78	74	59
Social functioning	78 (25)	92	73 (27)	87	85	81
Mental health	67 (18)	77	67 (18)	77	73	73
Health perception	46 (22)	72	48 (25)	60	60	59
Bodily pain	68 (28)	74	65 (31)	74	70	73
Energy	57 (18)	NA	NA	NA	NA	NA

In contrast to general HRQL questionnaires, disease-specific
questionnaires are only useful in specific populations of patients. They are
developed for use in clinical trials that request outcome measures
specifically tailored to a particular disease or intervention. They can also
detect small but clinically important changes over time or discriminate
between groups of patients with different disease severity.[62] General HRQL

questionnaires are often too broadly based and may contain items of little or no relevance for a specific disease. In addition, they may miss certain relevant items for a specific disease. For example, the MOS-24 does not include questions about visual functioning as a consequence of diplopia, which is very important for patients with Graves' ophthalmopathy. Therefore, the MOS-24 may be unable to measure small, but important changes in visual functioning over time. In the study of Gerding *et al.*[31] the MOS-24 could not discriminate between patients with mild or moderate Graves' ophthalmopathy.

Disease-specific questionnaires are available for many patient populations. Also, several vision-specific questionnaires were developed, such as the Visual Function Index (VFI),[67] the Activities of Daily Vision Scale (ADVS),[68] the Visual Activity Questionnaire (VAQ),[69] the VF-14,[70-72] the vision-related SIP (VR-SIP),[73,74] and the National Eye Institute-Visual Function Questionnaire (NEI-VFQ).[75] Most of these questionnaires were developed for patients with cataract, except for the VAQ and NEI-VFQ which were developed for a more general population of patients suffering from decreased visual acuity. Since Graves' ophthalmopathy patients generally do not suffer from decreased visual acuity but rather from diplopia, all of the above questionnaires are considered unsuitable as disease-specific HRQL measures for patients with Graves' ophthalmopathy. Although vision as well as diplopia can affect visual functioning, questionnaires like the VR-SIP or NEI-VFQ contain many scales or items within scales that are not relevant for patients with Graves' ophthalmopathy.

Therefore, a disease-specific HRQL questionnaire for patients with Graves' ophthalmopathy was recently developed (the Graves' Ophthalmopathy Quality Of Life questionnaire (GO-QOL),[56] to describe the HRQL and changes in HRQL over time as a consequence of GO disease and treatment. The questionnaire was developed in cooperation with patients to construct questions that are focused on functional (physical and psychosocial) limitations in daily life caused by Graves' ophthalmopathy that are important to patients and influence their quality of life. Sixteen questions were constructed to represent two different aspects of GO related to HRQL: A) Eight questions about problems with visual functioning as a consequence of double vision. Patients are asked to indicate the degree of impairment, because of their GO, in activities like driving, reading, watching TV, etc., during the past week, on a three-point Likert scale (not impaired, a little impaired, severely impaired). B) Eight questions about the psychosocial consequences of a changed appearance. Patients are asked to indicate how much they felt their appearance had changed, how much they felt they got unpleasant reactions from others, how much they felt the disease influenced their self-confidence and friendships, as a consequence of their GO, during the past week, also on a three-point Likert scale (strongly, a little bit, or not at all). All answers are scored from 1 to 3 points and then summarized to one total score for visual functioning and one total score for appearance. Both scores are transformed to a range from 0 to 100 points, a higher score indicating better health.

Three different studies were performed to pre-test, modify, and validate the GO-QOL. In the first study, based on 70 newly diagnosed patients with GO, the validity and internal consistency of the subscales were assessed.[56] Internal consistency (based on correlation of the items within a subscale) was high, indicating a good reliability of the subscales. Correlation between the two subscales and demographics, relevant clinical measures and general quality of life subscales from the MOS-24, supported the construct validity of the questionnaire. This means that the questionnaire is likely to measure what it is intended to measure, i.e. the impact of Graves' ophthalmopathy on visual and psychosocial functioning.

In a second study, the test-retest reliability of the GO-QOL was assessed in 89 consecutive patients visiting the outpatient clinic of the Orbital Center.[57] High correlation was found between the first and second completion of the questionnaire (with two weeks between surveys). A third study is now being carried out to assess the longitudinal validity and the efficiency of the questionnaire to detect clinically important differences in scores over time. A good reliability does not guarantee that the instrument can measure change in a clinical trial setting.[76] For the interpretation of, for example, treatment effects, it is also important to determine the amount of change in scores that constitutes an important difference in functioning for the patient. If the variability of this change between patients is relatively small, one can conduct clinical trials with relatively small sample sizes. The preliminary results of this study seem promising.

It can be concluded from these studies that the GO-QOL is a reliable and valid instrument to measure the impact of Graves' ophthalmopathy and its treatments on visual and psychosocial functioning in daily life. However, to be useful in studies in languages other than Dutch, the questionnaire needs to be translated and validated into different languages in a standardized way (using formal forward and backward translation methods) to guarantee the validity and reliability. A sound English translation of the GO-QOL is currently underway.

By measuring HRQL outcomes in a valid and standardized way, these outcomes can help to arrive at a better understanding of disease severity and the effects of treatment from the patients' point of view. This can be the first step to come towards an integrated view of disease severity and therapeutic outcome.

4.   REFERENCES

1. Van Dyk HJL. Orbital Graves' disease: a modification of the "NO SPECS" classification. Ophthalmology 1981; 88:479-483.
2. Morris JCI, Hay ID, Nelson RE, Jiang NS. Clinical utility of thyrotropin-receptor antibody assays: Comparison of radioreceptor and bioassay methods. Mayo Clin Proc 1988; 63:707-717.
3. Kahaly G, Schuler M, Sewell AC, Bernhard G, Beyer J, Krause U. Urinary glycosaminoglycans in Graves' ophthalmopathy. Clin Endocrinol 1990; 33:35-44.
4. Kahaly G, Stover C, Otto E, Beyer J, Schuler M. Glycosaminoglycans in thyroid-associated ophthalmopathy. Autoimmunity 1992; 13:81-88.
5. Kahaly G, Hansen C, Beyer J, Winand R. Plasma glycosaminoglycans in endocrine ophthalmopathy. J Endocrinol Invest 1994; 17:45-50.
6. Schuler M, Hansen C, Winand R, *et al.* Urinary and plasma glycosaminoglycans in endocrine ophthalmopathy. Dev Ophthalmol 1993; 25:58-67.
7. Feldon SE. Diagnostic tests and clinical techniques in the evaluation of Graves' ophthalmopathy. In: Wall JR, How J, eds. Graves' Ophthalmopathy. Oxford: Blackwell Scientific Publications. 1990, 79-93.
8. Prummel MF, Suttorp-Schulten MS, Wiersinga WM, Verbeek AM, Mourits MP, Koornneef L. A new ultrasonographic method to detect disease activity and predict response to immunosuppressive treatment in Graves ophthalmopathy. Ophthalmology 1993; 100:556-561.
9. Just M, Kahaly G, Higer HP, *et al.* M. Graves ophthalmopathy: role of MR imaging in radiation therapy. Radiology 1991; 179:187-190.
10. Utech CI, Khatibnia U, Winter PF, Wulle KG. MR T2 relaxation time for the assessment of retrobulbar inflammation in Graves' ophthalmopathy. Thyroid 1995; 5:185-193.
11. Hiromatsu Y, Kojima K, Ishisaka N, *et al.* Role of magnetic resonance imaging in thyroid-associated ophthalmopathy: its predictive value for therapeutic outcome of immunosuppressive therapy. Thyroid 1992; 2:299-305.
12. Hoh HB, Laitt RD, Wakeley C, *et al.* The STIR sequence MRI in the assessment of extraocular muscles in thyroid eye disease. Eye 1994; 8:506-510.
13. Chang TC, Kao SC, Huang KM. Octreotide and Graves' ophthalmopathy and pretibial myxoedema. Br Med J 1992; 304:158-158.
14. Durak I, Durak H, Ergin M, Yürekli Y, Kaynak S. Somatostatin receptors in the orbits. Clin Nucl Med 1995; 20:237-242.
15. Kahaly G, Diaz M, Hahn K, Beyer J, Bockisch A. Indium-111-pentetreotide scintigraphy in Graves' ophthalmopathy. J Nucl Med 1995; 36:550-554.
16. Kahaly G, Diaz M, Just M, Beyer J, Lieb W. Role of octreoscan and correlation with MR imaging in Graves' ophthalmopathy. Thyroid 1995; 5:107-111.
17. Mourits MP, Koornneef L, Wiersinga WM, Prummel MF, Berghout A, van der Gaag R. Clinical criteria for the assessment of disease activity in Graves' ophthalmopathy: A novel approach. Br J Ophthalmol 1989; 73:639-644.
18. Mourits MP, Prummel MF, Wiersinga WM, Koornneef L. Clinical activity score as a guide in the management of patients with Graves' ophthalmopathy. Clin Endocrinol 1997; 47:9-14.
19. Feldon SE, Weiner JM. Clinical significance of extraocular muscle volumes in Graves' ophthalmopathy. A quantitative computed tomography study. Arch Ophthalmol 1982; 100:1266-1269.

20. Feldon SE, Muramatsu S, Weiner JM. Clinical classification of Graves' ophthalmopathy. Identification of risk factors for optic neuropathy. Arch Ophthalmol 1984; 102:1469-1472.

21. Feldon SE, Lee CP, Muramatsu SK, Weiner JM. Quantitative computed tomography of Graves' ophthalmopathy. Arch Ophthalmol 1985; 103:213-215.

22. Hallin ES, Feldon SE. Graves' ophthalmopathy. II. Correlation of clinical signs with measures derived from computed tomography. Br J Ophthalmol 1988; 72:678-682.

23. Gorman CA. The measurement of change in Graves' ophthalmopathy. Thyroid 1998; 8:539-543.

24. Sullivan TJ, Kraft SP, Burack C, O'Reilly C. A functional scoring method for the field of binocular single vision. Ophthalmology 1992; 99:575-581.

25. Fells P, Kousoulides L, Pappa A, Munro P, Lawson J. Extraocular muscle problems in thyroid eye disease. Eye 1994; 8:497-505.

26. Mourits MP, Prummel MF, Wiersinga WM, Koornneef L. Measuring eye movements in Graves ophthalmopathy. Ophthalmology 1994; 101:1341-1346.

27. Gerling J, Lieb B, Kommerell G. Duction ranges in normal probands and patients with Graves' ophthalmopathy, determined using the Goldmann perimeter. Int Ophthalmol 1998; 21:213-221.

28. Rundle FF, Wilson CW. Measurement of duction movements of the eye. Clin Sci 1942; 4:385-399.

29. Demer JL, Kerman BM. Comparison of standardized echography with magnetic resonance imaging to measure extraocular muscle size. Am J Ophthalmol 1994; 118:351-361.

30. Guyatt GH, Feeny DH, Patrick DL. Measuring health related quality of life. Ann Intern Med 1993; 118:622-629.

31. Gerding MN, Terwee CB, Dekker FW, Prummel MF, Wiersinga WM. Quality of life in patients with Graves' ophthalmopathy is markedly decreased: measurement by the Medical Outcome Study Instrument. Thyroid 1997; 7.885-889.

32. Stewart AL, Hays RD, Ware JE. The MOS short-form general health survey: reliability and validity in a patient population. Med Care 1988; 26:724-735.

33. Wilson IB, Cleary PD. Linking clinical variables with health-related quality of life. JAMA 1995; 273:59-65.

34. Guyatt GH, Naylor D, Juniper E, Heyland DK, Jaeschke R, Cook DJ. Users' guides to the medical literature. XII. How to use articles about health-related quality of life. JAMA 1997; 277:1232-1237.

35. Testa MA, Simonson DC. Assessment of quality of life outcomes. N Engl J Med 1996; 334:835-840.

36. Classification of eye changes of Graves' disease. Thyroid 1992; 2:235-236.

37. Prummel MF, Mourits MP, Berghout A, *et al.* Prednisone and cyclosporine in the treatment of severe Graves' ophthalmopathy. N Engl J Med 1989; 321:1353-1359.

38. Baschieri L, Antonelli A, Nardi S, *et al.* Intravenous immunoglobulin versus corticosteroid in treatment of Graves' ophthalmopathy. Thyroid 1997; 7:579-585.

39. Mourits MP, van Kempen-Harteveld ML, Terwee CB, Koppeschaar HPF, Tick L. Randomized placebo-controlled study of radiotherapy for Graves' ophthalmopathy. VIth International Symposium on Graves' ophthalmopathy, Amsterdam, NL, November 27-28, 1998.

40. Prummel MF, Mourits MP, Blank L, Berghout A, Koornneef L, Wiersinga WM: Randomized double-blind trial of prednisone versus radiotherapy in Graves' ophthalmopathy. Lancet 1993; 342:949-954.

41. Khan JA, Doane JF, Whitacre MM. Does decompression diminish the discomfort of severe dysthyroid orbitopathy? Ophthal Plast Reconstr Surg 1995; 11:109-112.

42. Seegenschmiedt MH, Keilholz L, Gusek-Schneider G, *et al.* Endokrine orbitopathie: Vergleich der Langzeitergebnisse und Klassifikationen nach Radiotherapie. Strahlenther Onkol 1998; 174:449-456.

43. Kung AWC, Michon J, Tai KS, Chan FL. The effect of somatostatin versus corticosteroid in the treatment of Graves' ophthalmopathy. Thyroid 1996; 6:381-384.

44. Matejka G, Vergès B, Vaillant G, *et al.* Intravenous methylprednisolone pulse therapy in the treatment of Graves' ophthalmopathy. Horm Metab Res 1997; 30:93-98.

45. Bartalena L, Marcocci C, Bogazzi F, *et al.* Relation between therapy for hyperthyroidism and the course of Graves' ophthalmopathy. N Engl J Med 1998; 338:73-78.

46. Fatourechi V, Garrity JA, Bartley GB, Bergstralh EJ, Gorman CA. Orbital decompression in Graves' ophthalmopathy associated with pretibial myxedema. J Endocrinol Invest 1993; 16:433-437.

47. Fatourechi V, Bergstralh EJ, Garrity JA, *et al.* Predictors of response to transantral orbital decompression in severe Graves' ophthalmopathy. Mayo Clin Proc 1994; 69:841-848.

48. Fatourechi V, Garrity JA, Bartley GB, Bergstralh EJ, DeSanto LW, Gorman CA. Results of transantral orbital decompression performed primarily for cosmetic indications. Ophthalmology 1994; 101:938-942.

49. Garrity JA, Fatourechi V, Bergstralh EJ, *et al.* Results of transantral orbital decompression in 428 patients with severe Graves' ophthalmopathy. Am J Ophthalmol 1993; 116:533-547.

50. Bartley GB, Fatourechi V, Kadrmas EF, *et al.* Long-term follow-up of Graves' ophthalmopathy in an incidence cohort. Ophthalmology 1996; 103:958-962.

51. Linos DA, Karakitos D, Papademetriou J. Should the primary treatment of hyperthyroidism be surgical? Eur J Surg 1997; 163:651-657.

52. Olver JM: Botulinum toxin A treatment of overactive corrugator supercilii in thyroid eye disease. Br J Ophthalmol 1998; 82:528-533.

53. Paridaens D, Hans K, van Buitenen S, Mourits MP. The incidence of diplopia following coronal and translid orbital decompression in Graves' orbitopathy. Eye 1998; 12:800-805.

54. Tjon F, Sang M, Knegt P, *et al.* Transantral orbital decompression for Graves' disease. Clin Otolaryngol 1994; 19:290-294.

55. Törring O, Tallstedt L, Wallin G, *et al.* Graves' hyperthyroidism: treatment with antithyroid drugs, surgery, or radioiodine - a prospective, randomized study. J Clin Endocrinol Metab 1996; 81:2986-2993.

56. Terwee CB, Gerding MN, Dekker FW, Prummel MF, Wiersinga WM. Development of a disease-specific quality of life questionaire for patients with Graves' ophthalmopathy: the GO-QOL. Br J Ophthalmol 1998; 82:773-779.

57. Terwee CB, Gerding MN, Dekker FW, Prummel MF, van der Pol JP, Wiersinga WM. Test-retest reliability of the GO-QOL: A disease specific quality of life questionaire for patients with Graves' ophthalmopathy. J.Clin.Epidemiol. 1999(in press)

58. Kane RL, Maciejweski M, Finch M. The relationship of patient satisfaction with care and clinical outcomes. Med Care 1997; 35:714-730.

59. Guyatt GH, Jaeschke R, Feeny DH, Patrick DL. Measurement in clinical trials: Choosing the right approach. In: Spilker B, ed. Quality of life and pharmacoeconomics in clinical trials. Philadelphia: Lippincott-Raven Publishers, 1996, 41-48.

60. Schumacher M, Olschewski M, Schulgen G. Assessment of quality of life in clinical trials. Stat Med 1991; 10:1915-1930.

61. Streiner DL, Norman GR. Health Measurement Scales. A Practical Guide to Their Development and Use. Oxford: Oxford University Press, 1995.

62. Patrick DL, Deyo RA: Generic and disease-specific measures in assessing health status and quality of life. Med Care 1989; 27 (suppl 3):S217-S232,

63. Aaronson NK, Acquadro C, Alonso J, *et al.* International quality of life assessment (IQOLA) project. Quality of Life Research 1992; 1:349-351.

64. Ware JE, Sherbourne CD. The MOS 36-item Short-Form Health Survey (SF-36). I. Conceptual framework and item selection. Med Care 1992; 30:473-483.

65. Bergner M, Bobbitt RA, Kressel S, Pollard WE, Gilson BS, Morris JR. The Sickness Impact Profile: Conceptual formulation and methodology for the development of a health status measure. Int J Health Serv 1976; 6:393-415.

66. McEwen J. The Nottingham Health Profile. In: Walker SR, Rosser RM, eds. Quality of Life: Assessment and Application. Lancaster: MTP Press, 1988, 95.

67. Bernth-Petersen P. Visual functioning in cataract patients: methods of measuring and results. Acta Ophthalmol 1981; 59:198-205.

68. Mangione CM, Phillips RS, Seddon JM, *et al.* Development of the 'Actvities of Daily Vision Scale'. Med Care 1992; 30:1111-1126.

69. Sloane ME, Ball K, Owsley C, Bruni JR, Roenker DL. The visual activities questionnaire: developing an instrument for assessing problems in everyday visual tasks. Tech Dig Noninvasive AssessVis Sys 1992; 1:26-29.

70. Alonso J, Espallargues M, Andersen TF,*et al.* International applicability of the VF-14. An index of function in patients with cataracts. Ophthalmology 1997; 104:799-807.

71. Cassard SD, Patrick DL, Damiano AM, *et al.* Reproducibility and responsiveness of the VF-14. An index of functional impairment in patients with cataracts. Arch Ophthalmol 1995; 113:1508-1513.

72. Steinberg EP, Tielsch JM, Schein OD, *et al.* The VF-14. An index of functional impairment in patients with cataract. Arch Ophthalmol 1994; 112:630-638.

73. Desai P, Reidy A, Minassian DC, Vafidis G, Bolger J. Gains from cataract surgery: visual function and quality of life. Br J Ophthalmol 1996; 80:868-873.

74. Scott IU, Schein OD, West S, Bandeen-Roche K, Enger C, Folstein MF. Functional status and quality of life measurements among ophthalmic patients. Arch Ophthalmol 1994; 112:329-335.

75. NEI-VFQ Phase I Development Team. Measuring visual function: Test version of the National Eye Institute-Vision Function Questionnaire (NEI-VFQ). Santa Monica, California, RAND Corporation, 1995

76. Guyatt GH, Walter S, Norman G. Measuring change over time: Assessing the usefulness of evaluative instruments. J Chron Dis 1987; 40:171-178.

77. McNutt LC, Kaefring SL, Ossoinig KC. Echographic measurement of extraocular muscles. In: White D, Brown RE, eds. Ultrasound in Medicine. New York: Plenum Press, 1977, 927-932.

78. Ossoinig KC, Hermsen VM: Myositis of extraocular muscles diagnosed with standardized echography. In: Hillman JS, LeMay MM, eds. Ophthalmic Ultrasonography. The Hague: Dr. W. Junk, 1983, 381-392.

79. Willinsky RA, Arenson AM, Hurwitz JJ, Szalai J. Ultrasonic B-scan measurement of the extra-ocular muscles in Graves' orbitopathy. J Can Assoc Radiol 1984 35:171-173.

80. Given-Wilson R, Pope RM, Michell MJ, Cannon R, McGregor AM. The use of real-time orbital ultrasound in Graves' ophthalmopathy: a comparison with computed tomography. Br J Radiol 1989; 62:705-709.

81. Byrne SF, Gendron EK, Glaser JS, Feuer W, Atta H. Diameter of normal extraocular recti muscles with echography. Am J Ophthalmol 1991; 112:706-713.

82. Stewart AL, Greenfield S, Hays RD, *et al.* Functional status and well-being of patients with chronic conditions. Results from the Medical Outcomes Study. JAMA 1989; 262:907-913.

83. de Boer AGEM, Wijker W, Bartelsman JFW, deHaes HCJM. Inflammatory bowel diease questionnaire: Cross-cultural adaptation and further validation. Eur J Gastroenterol Hep 1995; 7:1043-1050.

Chapter 4

Assessment of disease activity of Graves' ophthalmopathy

Mark F. Prummel,* Wilmar M. Wiersinga, Maarten Ph. Mourits
*Department of Endocrinology, F5171, Academic Medical Center, University of Amsterdam, Meibergdreef 9, 1105 AZ Amsterdam, The Netherlands

The concept of disease activity originates from observations of the natural course of the eye signs in patients left untreated for the ophthalmopathy, and from a small number of histologic studies performed on orbital tissues from patients with variable duration of the eye disease.

1. NATURAL HISTORY

In 1923 ophthalmopathy patients were treated by "skillful neglect" and by "sending the patients to the country".[1] Nevertheless, Kessel *et al* noted that there was a tendency towards spontaneous regression of the eye signs over time, though without reaching the pre-morbid state.[1] These patients however were also left untreated for their hyperthyroidism, (which improved spontaneously as well), and no specific eye measurements were reported. Copper was one of the first authors to do specific measurements. He showed that the retrobulbar pressure, measured by an orbitonometer, decreased over time.[2] But it was Rundle who did sequential measurements in 12 patients who were not treated for the ophthalmopathy.[3] He followed these patients during 2½ years, recorded proptosis readings and measured the impairment of elevation using a vertometer.[4] He found that the eye disease begins with a dynamic phase, characterized by ingravescences and remissions, followed by a static phase: depicted as Rundle's curve (Fig. 1).[3] A similar curve was made by Dobyns (Fig. 2).[5] Both authors agreed that despite some remission, the eye disease often is still severe when the static phase is reached.[5,6]

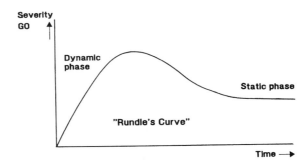

Figure 1. Rundle's curve, describing the natural course of the eye disease over a variable period of several months to a few years. (Contributed by M.F. Prummel)

Later studies have confirmed these early observations.[7] Perros *et al.* studied patients with mild ophthalmopathy and found that spontaneous improvement occurred in 64% of his 59 patients during a median follow-up of 12 months, while the disease remained stable in 22% and progressed in 14%.[8] Despite this high incidence of improvement, it is also clear that most

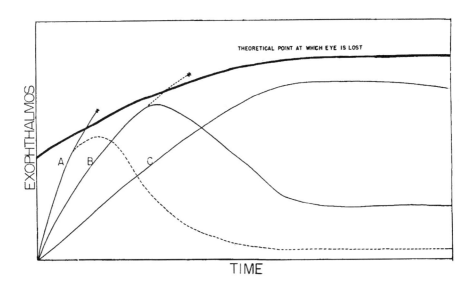

Figure 2. Schematic representation of the courses that progressive exophthalmos may follow. Heavy black line represents a theoretic point at which the eye may be lost. Proptosis, which develops over a long period of time, may become extreme without loss of the eye. Usually the longer the active process continues the more irreversible the proptosis becomes. At any time, the progress of the disease may abate and the eye recede as much as reversibility permits. (Reproduced with permission from the Publisher.[5])

patients think that their eyes never returned to normal: 54% (out of 120) in the study by Hamilton *et al.,*[9] and 61% (out of 120) in a study of Bartley *et al.,* with a median follow-up of 9½ years.[10]

Thus, most authors agree that the orbital disease starts with a period in which the disease gets worse: the active phase, in which there can be exacerbations and remissions up to a plateau is reached in which the disease is at its most severe stage. This plateau phase is then followed by a slow decrease in severity until a stable end-stage is reached: the inactive phase. However, often the eye signs and symptoms are still invalidating the patient.

Rundle's curve is generally accepted, despite the fact that the time axis is not clearly defined (Fig. 1): It is unclear how long it takes in individual patients before the stable end-stage is reached. This can take between several months to 5 years.[11] Even less is known about the pathogenesis of the transition from active into inactive disease. Here we will review the available histologic data pertaining to the distinction between active and burnt-out disease.

2. HISTOLOGY DURING ACTIVE AND INACTIVE DISEASE

Naffziger operated on a number of patients with very severe, "malignant" ophthalmopathy and found edematous tissue in patients with early disease, whereas those with longer standing ophthalmopathy had much fibrous tissue.[12] In the early stages he found just swelling of the muscle fibers, during the "intermediate" stages a mononuclear cell infiltrate was observed, while in the late stages dense collagen scar tissue was prominent.[12] Dunnington and Berke summarized their biopsy examinations also as the occurrence of a lymphocytic infiltrate, marked edema of muscle fibers, and fibrosis.[13] Russell Brain contrasted histologic examinations in patients with short duration of disease (lymphocytic and plasma cell infiltrates, edema) to the findings at autopsy of a patient who had suffered from Graves' ophthalmopathy for 6½ years.[14] In this patient he saw massive fibrosis with the globe appearing to be anchored to the orbit by dense fibrous tissue strands. The eye muscles could only be identified as thin fibrotic bands. Daicker reported a chronic lymphocytic infiltration, edema, and fibroblast activation in the biopsies from early, active patients, whereas in patients with longstanding ophthalmopathy only fibrosis and fat accumulation was seen.[15] He also observed that the eye muscles could actually be more enlarged in inactive, than in active patients, and suggested that corticosteroids or radiotherapy are only effective during the active phase of fibroblast activation. Other studies have also noted the coexistence of a lymphocytic infiltrate with fibroblasts and so-called "young connective tissue".[5,16-18] Tallstedt and Norberg found fibrosis, collagen deposition and activated fibroblasts in 4 patients with apparently inactive disease, whereas these abnormalities were also seen in a patient with rapidly progressive disease in whom, however, a more marked lymphocytic infiltrate was found.[19]

Thus, the few histologic studies published do support the concept of Rundle's curve. During the active stage there usually is edema, a lymphocytic infiltrate and activation of fibroblasts. In the end-stages, there is only fibrosis. It follows that to discriminate on histology between active and inactive disease, the presence of fibrosis is not helpful, since it is present throughout the disease process. One has to rely on the detection of edema and a lymphocytic infiltrate, which is however usually localized and its detection is thus liable to sampling errors.

3.   DISEASE ACTIVITY: CLINICAL IMPLICATIONS

Daicker was the first to suggest that medical treatment (radiotherapy, corticosteroids) will only be effective during the active phases.[15] For, both treatments are immunosuppressive and anti-inflammatory and will thus act on the lymphocytic infiltrate and edema of the active phase, and it is highly unlikely that they will improve the fibrous scar tissue left in the end-stages. However, end-stage ophthalmopathy can still cause considerable proptosis and diplopia, and this kind of patients will therefore seek help in specialized clinics. These inactive patients will probably not benefit from immunosuppresion and should undergo rehabilitative surgery. Whereas a patient with the same degree of proptosis and diplopia in the active phase can be treated with steroids or irradiation, and surgery at that time might actually be harmful because the ongoing immune process may reverse the surgical result.

Thus, the implications of the concept of disease activity are that the stage of the disease rather than the severity should dictate whether to use medical therapy or surgery. Obviously, this can be easy. A patient with rapidly progressive ophthalmopathy of six months duration will be treated medically. In contrast, a patient with diplopia, finally referred after 10 years, will be scheduled immediately for squint surgery. However, in many patients with Graves' ophthalmopathy this is much less obvious, and then an assessment of the activity might be helpful to decide on their treatment.

The concept of disease activity might also explain the fact that whichever medical treatment is given, only about two-thirds of the patients will respond.[20] For, in most studies patients are recruited on the basis of the severity of their eye disease. Implying, that both active and inactive patients with similar severity are subjected to a medical treatment that will only benefit the active patients. If we were able to restrict our medical treatment to active patients only, the response rate to these therapies might increase considerably.

In conclusion, assessing the stage of the disease in individual patients will help us to decide on the most appropriate and logical therapy. Which is why many different groups have tried to develop methods to assess disease activity. Each of these parameters should however be validated.

4.   VALIDATION OF ACTIVITY PARAMETERS

It is not easy to assess whether a given parameter of disease activity actually reflects a lymphocytic infiltrate, edema and fibroblast activation. The proper control for this would be to relate the parameter to a biopsy of extraocular muscles, or maybe connective tissue. For obvious reasons this approach is not feasible, because such a biopsy might be damaging to the patient. In addition, the biopsy would be liable to sampling error as described above. Thus the value of an activity parameter can not easily be related to a gold standard. Consequently we have to do with a surrogate standard.

The surrogate criterion to be met by an activity parameter is its value in predicting the outcome of immunosuppressive treatment. Why? Since the underlying concept is that the lymphocytic infiltrate *etc* of the active phase is amenable to medical intervention, an activity marker that is reflecting this ongoing immune process would be able to predict a beneficial response to immunosuppressive therapies. On the other hand, if an activity marker reflects fibrotic scar tissue this parameter would predict a negative outcome of immunosuppression. In other words if a marker has a high positive predictive value (+ve PV) for response to medical treatment, it detects the active patients. An activity marker with high negative predictive value (-ve PV; predicting no response) would be indicative of inactive burnt-out disease.

When there is good basic evidence that a marker of disease activity might reflect activity, this marker should then be tested against the (surrogate) standard: the clinical outcome of treatment. Using a two-by-two table (Fig.3) sensitivity, specificity, +ve PV and -ve PV can be calculated, indicating the clinical usefulness of the proposed test. One should however remember that this is a surrogate standard and subject to various confounding factors. Thus, the performance of a test will also depend on the way the clinical outcome is measured, on the efficacy of the treatment, and on the natural history of the disease. Since no treatment is always effective, the +ve PV will never be

100%. Also, because spontaneous improvement can occur during the beginning of the inactive phase, the -ve PV will never be 100% as well. Lastly, even genetic factors might influence treatment outcome; several HLA markers have been shown to indicate good or bad response to medical therapy.[21,22]

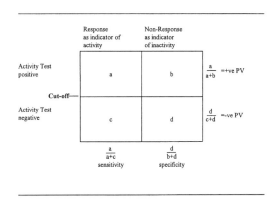

Figure 3. Validation of a test determining disease activity. The test is performed at base-line, and the test result is compared to the response to immunosuppressive treatment (usually after six months). A cut-off is best determined by a Receiver-Operator-Characteristics curve.

Now we will review the different parameters for disease activity, and whether they have been tested in the above explained fashion. We will start with purely clinical parameters, then focus on imaging techniques, and finally on serum markers.

5.   CLINICAL PARAMETERS

The most obvious clinical parameter is the duration of the eye disease. Ophthalmopathy of really short duration should by default be active, extremely long standing complaints should be due to inactive disease. However, as stated above the duration of active ophthalmopathy is extremely variable (anywhere between several months to five years), and it is indeed the experience of most investigators that the mean duration of the eye disease is similar in responding and non-responding patients.[23,24] Still, Donaldson *et al.* did find a correlation between the response to prednisone and the duration of the *exacerbation* of the eye signs.[25] It is maybe remarkable that nobody has actually reported a 2x2 table analyzing its clinical usefulness. However, we have tried to compile the individual patient data of two published papers from Pisa resulting in the data depicted in Fig. 4.[26,27]

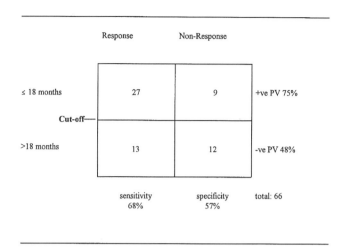

Figure 4. The value of the duration of the eye disease in predicting the outcome of immunosuppression. Patient data were compiled from two Italian studies.

A second approach would be to just observe the patient over time. When there is progression, the disease is active; when the eye signs are stable, the process is inactive. This approach has several drawbacks. First, in active patients seeking help effective therapy is postponed. Secondly, this concept heavily leans on the power of our measurements to detect significant changes in disease severity. This power is certainly limited: significant changes in Hertel has been said to be 2 mm, but inter-observer variation is considerable.[28] In our own experience detectable changes in 2 months occur seldomly, also in patients who had a very successful course of steroids (see below).

Trying to determine the activity of the eye disease by clinical examination is not new. Van Dyke proposed the mnemonic RELIEF,[29] and in 1981 Sergott *et al.* included clinical parameters in their activity score.[30] None of these indexes were tested in a prospective study. In 1989 a Clinical Activity Score (CAS) was proposed,[31] which is based on the classical signs of inflammation: *dolor, rubor, tumor, functio laesa* (the fifth sign *calor*, heat, was considered but found unfeasible to measure; see Table 1). The CAS has one draw-back: for the impaired function part observation during two months is necessary. Although the occurrence of a change in two months is relatively low (proptosis, 19%; motility, 7%; visual acuity, 2%), these signs do have a high +ve PV and are needed in the CAS. In the first, but retrospective analysis of the CAS, its performance was good.[31] It was then tested in formal prospective study with the following results: CAS ≥4 had a +ve PV of 80%, but a -ve PV of 64%.[32] Thus, although it is still a useful and simple test, it cannot be used on its own to decide to perform surgery directly.[33,34]

Table 1. The 10 items of the Clinical Activity Score (CAS). For each item, one point is given. The sum of these points is the CAS.

Item		Description
Pain	1	Painful, oppressive feeling on or behind the globe, during the last 4 weeks
	2	Pain on attempted up-, side-, or down-gaze
Redness	3	Redness of the eye lids
	4	Diffuse redness of the conjunctiva, covering at least one quadrant
Swelling	5	Swelling of the eyelid(s)
	6	Chemosis
	7	Swollen caruncle
	8	Increase in proptosis of 2 mm or more during a period of 1-3 months
Impaired function	9	Decrease of eye movements in any direction of 5 degrees or more during a period of 1-3 months
	10	Decrease of visual acuity of 1 line or more on the Snellen chart (using a pinhole) during a period of 1-3 months

6.   IMAGING TECHNIQUES

6.1   Magnetic Resonance Imaging (MRI)

MRI does not use ionizing irradiation but a very strong magnetic field to line up the protons (hydrogen atoms) in the body. Protons can be viewed as small magnetic bars with a north and south pole, which spin (actually wobble) around an axis, and by applying a gradient magnetic field the axes of the spins are lined up.[35] Radiofrequency pulses from a radiofrequency transmitter coil (an antenna) bring the protons in a higher energy state, which will shift their spinning axes creating a radiofrequency field that can be detected by a receiver coil. The signal thus detected depends on the proton density of the tissue, and the T1 and T2 relaxation times of the tissues. The T1 time represents the rate at which the excited protons realign with the magnetic field. The T2 relaxation time represents another characteristic of the tissues. It is not determined by the axis of the spinning proton, but by the phase of the spin. The radiowave will also bring all spinning protons into the same phase (all north poles are pointing in the same direction). When the pulse is switched off, the protons start to dephase at a rate which is called the T2 relaxation time.[35]

Especially the T2 weighted images have been found useful to detect edema and inflammation in extraocular eye muscles on MRI. Just *et al* described that a long T2 time in the eye muscles before treatment were associated with a good response to orbital irradiation.[36] This first report were followed by others who confirmed that the T2 time decreases after immuno-suppressive therapy.[37,38] This suggests a transition from an edematous, inflammatory phase into a fibrotic end-stage. Indeed, Laitt *et al* found a correlation with the Clinical Activity Score and T2 times, using a more sophisticated protocol which suppresses the fat signal (short tau inversion recovery, STIR).[39] Until now only one study assessed the value of T2 time measurements to predict the outcome of immunosuppressive treatment (intravenous steroids).[40] In this small study in 23 patients, a +ve PV of 69% and a -ve PV of 86% was found.

Thus, MRI seems a promising method to detect disease activity, but the good -ve PV should be confirmed in a larger study.

6.2 Octreotide scintigraphy

Octreotide is an eight amino acid analog of the 14-aminoacid neuropeptide somatostatin with a more prolonged half-life of 2-3 hours compared to the 2-3 min half-life of native somatostatin. Somatostatine serves as neurotransmitter and as a hormone by interacting with different G-protein coupled somatostatin receptors widely distributed throughout the body. Octreotide can be radiolabeled and [^{111}In-DTPA-D-Phe^1] octreotide is used in nuclear medicine to visualize tissues with somatostatin receptors. Postema *et al.* were the first to show pronounced orbital octreotide uptake in patients with Graves' ophthalmopathy.[41] The amount of octreotide uptake correlates positively with the Clinical Activity Score,[41,42] and with the above mentioned T2 relaxation time.[43] In inactive patients the octreotide accumulation is weak and resembles the uptake in normal orbits.[44] The cause of the orbital uptake of octreotide is unknown, but it is hypothesized that activated lymphocytes, or fibroblasts express somatostatin receptors.[45]

Octreotide scanning of the orbits is usually done at 4 hours after injection and the later 24 hours imaging is probably not very useful.[42,46,47] The administered dose in the earlier studies was 22 Mbq (16 mSv, a radiation dose similar to that of a chest CT scan), but others have used approximately half of that dose and could still obtain a good image.[42,47] Uptake in the orbit should be corrected for background blood pool radioactivity, which can be done using the temporal skull, although we found the occipital skull to be a better correction for background uptake.[47]

Octreotide uptake measurements can be used to predict the outcome to immunosuppression.[48] In a small, preliminary study with 12 patients Krassas *et al* found a +ve PV of 100%, and a -ve PV of 83%.[49] We studied a group of 22 patients and found a +ve PV of 92%, and a -ve PV of 70%.[47]

Whether octreotide scintigraphy deserves a place in the diagnostic work-up of ophthalmopathy patients remains to be seen, and results from larger studies are expected soon. However, it is an expensive diagnostic tool with a not negligible radioactivity burden.

6.3   Ultrasound

Ultrasound is an inexpensive method to visualize the orbital contents and has been used to measure the thickness of the eye muscles.[50] However, it can also depict the internal echogenecity of the eye muscles which is best done using two-dimensional A-mode echography (Fig. 5).

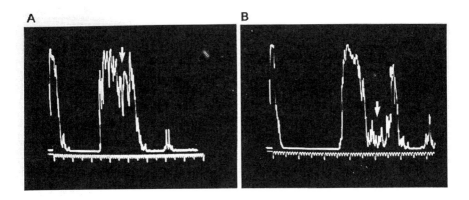

Figure 5. Characteristic example of A-mode ultrasonography in a patient with inactive (A), and active (B) ophthalmopathy. Note the irregular, and high reflectivity pattern in the eye muscle of patient A, as opposed to the low reflectivity in patient B.[51]

We found, that the internal reflectivity of the soundbeam is low in patients with active eye disease, presumably due to edema, whereas the reflectivity is high and irregular in inactive patients, due to fibrotic echogenic scar tissue.[51] In our preliminary study in 16 patients the method seemed promising: +ve PV, 73%; -ve PV 100%.[51] However, we have now tested this method in 56 patients with moderately severe ophthalmopathy, and the results were rather disappointing (+ve PV: 85%; -ve PV: 60%). Although the imaging technique is inexpensive, it is not easy to perform and is rather operator dependent. A-mode ultrasonography alone is thus not very helpful, although it might be a good adjunct tool in combination with other parameters for disease activity.

7.   LABORATORY MEASUREMENTS

A key difference between the active and inactive phase of Graves' ophthalmopathy is the lymphocytic infiltrate present in the orbital tissues during the active stage only. The characteristics of this infiltrate are discussed in Chapter 2, but in short we know that the lymphocytes produce cytokines. These cytokines can stimulate GAG production by fibroblasts, upregulate adhesion molecules and other immunomodulatory molecules like HSP72 and HLA-DR. Measurements of these cytokines, their soluble receptors or of the molecules they upregulate in serum might potentially differentiate the active from the inactive stage. However, there are some drawbacks to this approach. First, many of these molecules are also involved in Graves' thyroid disease, which might hinder their utility to detect activity of the Graves' eye disease. Secondly, the volume of orbital tissues is rather small and even if orbital cytokines are released into the bloodstream their presumably small quantity might be difficult to detect. Thirdly, cytokines in serum are to a large extent bound to soluble receptors, carrier proteins and even autoantibodies, which all can block the epitopes for the antibodies used in sandwich immunoassays which will therefore not measure all the cytokines present.[52] Here we will review the activity parameters related to the lymphocytic infiltrate in the orbit.

7.1   Lymphocyte function tests in peripheral blood

Sergott *et al.* measured sheep-erythrocyte Rosette formation by peripheral blood lymphocytes from patients with Graves' ophthalmopathy and related the result to the outcome of steroid treatment. They found that the responsive (active) patients had a significantly decreased percentage of rosette formation.[53] The number of spontaneous rosette-forming cells increases upon corticosteroid treatment in the responding patients, reaching values comparable to inactive and normal controls.[30] Similar results were obtained by other investigators,[22,54] but to our knowledge, presently this test is not used anymore for predicting outcome of immunosuppression.

7.2   Serum cytokine levels

The first "cytokine" measured was the Migration Inhibition Factor (MIF).[55,56] Van der Gaag *et al* found that MIF was present in 11/18 (61%) clinically active ophthalmopathy patients, compared to only 2/14 (14%; p=0.008) inactive patients.[57] However, the MIF is measured in a rather cumbersome bioassay. Nowadays highly sensitive sandwich ELISAs are being used to detect a fast growing number of cytokines.

Activated lymphocytes express IL-2 receptors and release a truncated form of this protein called the soluble IL-2 Receptor (sIL-2R). sIL-2R levels were found to be elevated in patients with severe ophthalmopathy,[58] and this correlates with disease activity.[59] However, the clinical usefulness of sIL-2R levels is limited with a +ve PV of only 71%, and -ve PV of 54%.[59] IL-6 is produced by lymphocytes, but also by fibroblasts and tumor cells and is elevated in serum from patients with Graves' hyperthyroidism.[60] Its soluble receptor (sIL-6R) is elevated in hyperthyroidism, but was also found to be related to the activity of the ophthalmopathy.[60] However, because of the huge overlap in sIL-6R values between active and inactive ophthalmopathy patients it is unlikely to be helpful to diagnose activity in individual patients. CD30 is a protein expressed on the membrane of activated T-helper 2 cells, and a soluble form (sCD30) released by proteolytic cleavage can be measured in serum. It was found to be elevated in patients with active Graves' thyroid disease, correlating with the titer of TSH-R antibodies.[61] It is unknown whether ophthalmopathy might be another determinant of sCD30 levels.

IL-1 is a potent stimulator of GAG production by fibroblasts, and this can be inhibited by IL-1 Receptor antagonist and by the soluble IL-1 receptor (sIL-1R).[62] The soluble form of the IL-1 receptor antagonist (sIL-1RA) and the sIL-1R can be measured in serum, and it was hypothesized that higher levels of these IL-1 inhibitors would protect the patient with ophthal-mopathy.[63] Indeed, it was shown that patients who responded well to radiotherapy had higher baseline sIL-1R and sIL-1RA levels than those who did not respond. Also, in the responders a significant increase in these levels occurred after radiotherapy, which did not occur in the nonresponders.[63] The predictive values of sIL-1R and sIL-1RA were not reported, but the authors also found that the levels of these IL-1 inhibitors were lower in smoking than in non-smoking patients.[63] During the symposium one presentation reported that smoking (an important risk factor for Graves' ophthalmopathy), is an important confounder in the interpretation of cytokine levels. Both in ophthalmopathy patients and in healthy controls serum levels of IL-1RA, sIL-2R, IL-6, sIL-6R, TNFαR-I and TNFαR-II, and sCD30 were significantly higher in smokers as compared to non-smokers. None of these cytokines could actually predict the response to retrobulbar irradiation.

Until now no single cytokine was found to reliably predict the outcome of immunosuppression. Cytokines act in a network, and this network might regulate itself through other cytokines. It might well be that we would have to measure a number of different cytokines, or a ratio of "stimulating" to "inhibitory" cytokines to get an impression of the activity of a disease. However, 'new' cytokines are still discovered and it might be worthwhile to evaluate them also. Nevertheless, the already investigated cytokines are known to cause a number of secondary effects (see above) and for the purpose of detecting disease activity, one might also look at these secondary events.

7.3   Immunomodulatory molecules

As explained in Chapter 1, cytokines and other factors (including immunoglobulins) have been shown to upregulate various adhesion molecules on orbital fibroblasts. Adhesion molecules play an important role in directing the traffic of circulating lymphocytes towards their target: homing.[64,65] ICAM-1 is such an adhesion molecule abundantly present in orbital tissue of active ophthalmopathy patients.[66,67] Soluble forms of ICAM-1 (sICAM-1) are shedded into the circulation and might therefore reflect the expression of ICAM-1 in the orbit. Indeed, Heufelder and Bahn found elevated levels of sICAM-1 in sera of patients with active eye disease (compared to patients with no, or inactive ophthalmopathy) and found that sICAM-1 levels decrease upon prednisone treatment.[68] Their findings were recently confirmed by De Bellis *et al.*,[69] who showed that patients with active ophthalmopathy had significantly increased levels of sICAM-1, although Graves' hyperthyroid disease patients without eye involvement also had higher levels than controls, albeit still lower than the ophthalmopathy patients. This might be due to the fact that ICAM-1 is expressed in thyroid tissue as well as in orbital tissues in Graves' disease. Another adhesion molecule, ELAM-1 is found in orbital tissues but not in the thyroid and the same group reported clearly elevated sELAM-1 levels in ophthalmopathy patients, but not in patients with Graves' thyroid disease without eye involvement.[69] According to their data, there was even no overlap between sELAM-1 levels in ophthalmopathy patients and hyperthyroidism patients, and the levels had a nice correlation with the CAS (r=0.55; P<0.002).[69] Another molecule upregulated by cytokines in orbital tissue is HSP-72, which is a super-antigen able to induce an autoantibody response. Indeed, anti-HSP72 antibodies have been found in sera from patients with Graves' disease, but the levels did not correlate with disease activity.[70] Serum HSP72 levels have not been measured in Graves' disease patients.

7.4   Autoantibodies

Since we do not know the antigen responsible for the autoimmune attack in the orbit, disease specific autoantibodies cannot be measured yet. There was some hope that antibodies against a 64 kDa eye muscle protein might reflect the activity of the eye disease, but we now know that it is not an eye muscle specific protein and that 20 % of normal controls also have anti-64 kDa autoantibodies, and the value of determining these antibodies has been questioned seriously.[71] Recent evidence for the presence of the TSH-R in the orbit, has given new life to the old hypothesis that TSH-R autoantibodies might in fact cross-react with the thyroid and orbit and be the link for the two manifestations of Graves' disease. Patients with ophthalmopathy indeed have higher levels of TSH-R autoantibodies,[72] but in older studies they do not seem to correlate with clinical characteristics of the eye disease.[73] In the Symposium, one presentation reported a very good correlation between stimulating TSH-R autoantibodies and the Clinical Activity Score.

7.5   Glycosaminoglycans (GAG)

GAGs play a key role in the manifestations of Graves' ophthalmopathy. They are hydrophilic proteoglycans which attract water and are the main reason for the increase in the volume of orbital tissues.[74] They are produced by activated fibroblasts,[75] and therefore GAGs might serve as a marker of active eye disease. GAGs are present in plasma and urine also in healthy controls, and are thus not specific for Graves' ophthalmopathy. In a recent study, Pappa *et al* found no correlation between serum hyaluronan levels and hyaluronan tissue levels.[74] Nevertheless, Kahaly *et al* found that ophthalmopathy patients have higher urinary GAG levels compared to controls and to patients with Graves' hyperthyroidism without eye disease.[76] Though there was a considerable overlap, they could find a cut-off value that could discriminate active from inactive patients (assessed on clinical criteria): +ve PV 68%, -ve PV 96%. Others could, however, not confirm their findings and found similar urinary GAG excretion in ophthalmopathy patients and controls.[77] In later studies the group of Kahaly used a HPLC method to determine GAG levels, which improved the biochemical analysis considerably.[78] Using this method, they again found higher levels of GAG excretion in active patients compared to inactive patients.[79] They also reported significantly elevated plasma GAG levels in patients with active, untreated ophthalmopathy, whereas plasma GAG levels were normal in patients with treated, inactive eye disease.[80] However, a formal prospective study using the 'gold' standard of the therapeutic outcome after immunosuppression has not yet been published.

8. COMBINATION OF PARAMETERS FOR DISEASE ACTIVITY

From Table 2 it is clear that none of the activity parameters can be used alone to make the therapeutic decision whether it is worthwhile to administer immunosuppression, or whether it is safe to perform rehabilitative surgery. Most parameters have a rather good +ve PV, but bad -ve PV, and only the MRI or the urinary GAG excretion hold a promise to be able to detect inactive disease (e.g. have a good -ve PV). However, these latter tests still need confirmation in a larger prospective study, and it is unlikely that a single test will accurately indicate disease activity. We feel, that we will need a combination of tests to optimize the discrimination between active and inactive disease.

Table 2. Validation of various activity parameters by their accurate prediction of outcome of immunosuppressive therapy.

Activity parameter	Cut off	+ve PV	-ve PV	N	Ref
Clinical					
Duration of GO	18 months	75	48	61	26,27
CAS	4	80	64	43	32
Imaging techniques					
MRI	1.8	69	86	23	40
Octreoscan	1.85	92	70	22	47
Ultrasound	30 %	85	60	56	--
Laboratory measurements					
sIL-2 R	650 U/ml	71	54	47	59
Urinary GAG's	25 mg/24 hrs	(68)	(96)	72	76

+ve PV, positive predictive value; -ve PV, negative predictive value; N, number of patients. Urinary GAG's were tested against the CAS.

This is not as simple as one might think. Let us consider two hypothetical patients with a similar severity of their Graves' ophthalmopathy (Table 3). In these patients a number of items indicating disease activity have been assessed, and in both patients three are positive, indicating that they might respond to immunosuppression. However, both also have three items that indicate that they might go to surgery without prior immunosuppression. Obviously, some items might have a better prognostic value and should have a bigger weight in assessing the activity status. How can we establish the relative impact of the items? Also considering that some of these parameters are expensive (octreotide scan, MRI).

Table 3. Results of various activity tests in two patients with similar disease severity, with the respective cut-off values.

Activity parameter	Patient 1	Patient 2	Cut-off used
Total Eye Score	12	12	-
Duration of GO (years)	½	5	1½
CAS (0-7)	3	5	4
Ultrasound (%)	45	10	30
Octreoscan (uptake ratio)	2.50	1.30	1.85
GAG excretion (mg/24 hr)	20	80	25
MRI (signal intensity ratio)	2.5	1.4	1.9
Items indicating response	3	3	
Items indicating no response	3	3	
Response	?	?	

To find which set of weighted activity parameters is useful in predicting response to immunosuppression we performed a study in 66 patients with moderately severe ophthalmopathy (defined as proptosis >25 mm, and/or restricted eye muscle motility quantified using a motility meter[81]). In these patients various parameters of disease activity were measured at baseline, after which they were subjected to retrobulbar irradiation. The response to this radiotherapy was assessed six months after the treatment using predefined criteria. Out of 66 patients, 35 (53%) responded and 31 (47%) did not. We then analyzed whether any of the activity parameters could predict this response on its own, and in agreement with the above mentioned reports (Table 2) found that none of them could. With the help of the Department of Clinical Epidemiology and Biostatistics, the individual data were entered in a multivariate logistic regression analysis model to weigh the relative impact of each parameter on the prediction of response to radiotherapy. The first to be entered in the model were the inexpensive parameters (e.g. duration of disease, CAS), followed by laboratory and imaging results.

As a first example we here show the outcome of such a model using a very limited number of eye disease parameters: Duration, severity (assessed by the Total Eye Score), Clinical Activity Score, ultrasound and octreoscan. Using this input, the model actually results in a so-called "Response Score" = 0.5 (duration in yrs) + 0.2 (TES) -0.05 (US) + 1.01 (OC ratio) +7

Using this model a Response Score could be calculated in 66 patients. A high score of >9 had a +ve PV of 78%, a -ve PV of 64%, with an AUC of 0.81, which is indeed somewhat better than the corresponding figures for the single tests. We feel that such a score will become a better predictor of response once other parameters (MRI, urinary GAG, or sELAM-1) are added. Is this still helpful in daily clinical practice? Let us consider the example of Table 3 and now add the formula from the computer model (Table 4). As can be seen, the model results in high "response score" in patient one, and in low score in the non-responding patient 2.

Table 4. Activity test results in the two patients of Table 3 weighted by using the "Response Score"

Test	Patient 1	Response Score	Patient 2	Response Score
Duration of GO	½	-0.25	1½	-2.5
TES	12	+2.40	12	+2.40
US	10	-0.50	45	-2.25
Octreoscan	2.50	+2.53	1.30	+1.31
		+7		+7
Response score		9.43		.70

There are some drawbacks to this solution in combining different parameters. First, the model would have to be tested in patient groups with varying degrees of severity, and second it might be dependent on the kind of treatment given.

9. CONCLUSION

The concept of disease activity is generally accepted, and the implications (e.g. the prediction of response to immunosuppression) of the concept are clear. However, it has proven to be difficult to assess in which stage the disease is in an individual patients, except in very obvious cases such as malignant ophthalmopathy. Why would that be?

First of all, we do not have a "gold standard" to assess the reliability of a given activity parameter. The "surrogate standard" (response to immunosuppression) is not as robust as one might think. Secondly, the various parameters might actually represent different aspects of the disease. For instance, edema might be measurable by ultrasound or MRI, whereas a lymphocytic infiltrate without much edema might not be detected by the imaging techniques. The levels of sELAM-1 might reflect the lymphocytic infiltrate, but not the edema. Thirdly, the disease activity might actually differ in the various muscles (or tissues) within one patient, resulting in ambiguous test results. Fourthly, we are still hindered by the fact that the cause of Graves' ophthalmopathy is still unknown, and that we have to rely on activity tests which are not specific for the orbital disease. For instance, sICAM-1 levels are also influenced by the thyroidal disease. The presence of edema might not always be caused by an active lymphocytic infiltrate, but also by venous obstruction due to long-standing swelling of the eye muscles.

Should we therefore abandon the quest for a reliable disease activity test? We think not. The implications at stake are big enough: rehabilitative surgery, or immunosuppression. On the contrary, the above mentioned problems imply that we need a combination of (preferably inexpensive) tests. We have shown that weighing different activity parameters is possible and feasible.

10.   REFERENCES

1. Kessel L, Hyman HT, Lande H. A study of fifty consecutive cases of exophthalmic goiter. Arch Int Med 1923; 31: 433-454.
2. Copper AC. An introduction to clinical orbitonometry. Thesis University of Leiden 1948;
3. Rundle FF. Development and course of exophthalmos and ophthalmoplegia in Graves' disease with special reference to the effect of thyroidectomy. Cli Sci 1945; 5: 177-194.
4. Rundle FF. Management of exophthalmos and related ocular changes in Graves' disease. Metabolism 1957; 6: 36-48.
5. Dobyns BM. Present concepts of the pathologic physiology of exopthalmos. J Clin Endocrinol Metab 1950; 10: 1202-1230.
6. Rundle FF. Ocular changes in Graves' disease. Q J Med 1960; 29: 113-126.
7. Streeten DHP, Anderson GH, Reed GF, Woo P. Prevalence, natural history and surgical treatment of exophthalmos. Clin Endocrinol 1987; 27: 125-133.
8. Perros P, Crombie AL, Kendall-Taylor P. Natural history of thyroid associated ophthalmopathy. Clin Endocrinol 1995; 42: 45-50.
9. Hamilton HE, Schultz RO, De Gowin EL. The endocrine eye lesion in hyperthyroidism. Arch Int Med 1960; 105: 675-685.
10. Bartley GB, Fatourechi V, Kadrmas EF, *et al*. Long-term follow-up of Graves Ophthalmopathy in an incidence cohort. Ophthalmology 1996; 103: 958-962.
11. Burch H, Wartofsky L. Graves' ophthalmopathy: Current concepts regarding pathogenesis and management. Endocr Rev 1993; 14: 747-793.
12. Naffziger HC. Pathologic changes in the orbit in progressive exophthalmos. Arch Ophthalmol 1933; 9: 1-12.
13. Dunnington JH, Berke RN. Exophthalmos due to chronic orbital myositis. Arch Ophthalmol 1943; 30: 446-466.
14. Brain RW. Exophthalmic ophthalmoplegia. Q J Med 1938; 31: 293-323.
15. Daicker B. Das gewebliche Substrat der verdickten ausseren Augenmuskeln bei der endokrinen Orbitopathie. Klin Mbl Augenheilk 1979; 174: 843-847.
16. Rundle FF, Finlay-Jones LR, Noad KB. Malignant exophthalmos: a quantitative analysis of the orbital tissues. Australasian Ann Med 1953; 2: 1-8.

17. Hufnagel TJ, Hickey WF, Cobbs WH, Jakobiec FA, Iwamoto T, Eagle RC. Immunohistochemical and ultrastrucural studies on the exenterated orbital tissues of a patient with Graves' disease. Ophthalmology 1984; 91: 1411-1419.

18. Kroll AJ, Kuwabara T. Dysthyroid ocular myopathy. Arch Ophthalmol 1966; 76: 244-257.

19. Tallstedt L, Norberg R. Immunohistochemical staining of normal and Graves' extraocular muscle. Inv Ophthalmol Vis Sc 1988; 29: 175-184.

20. Gayno JP, Strauch G. Cyclosporine and Graves' ophthalmopathy. Horm Res 1987; 26: 190-197.

21. Van der Gaag R, Wiersinga WM, Koornneef L, *et al.* HLA-DR4 associated response to corticosteroids in Graves' ophthalmopathy patients. J Endocrinol Invest 1990; 13: 489-492.

22. Preus M, Frecker MF, Stenszky V, Balazs C, Farid NR. A prognostic score for Graves' disease. Clin Endocrinol 1985; 23: 653-661.

23. Prummel MF, Mourits MP, Berghout A, *et al.* Prednisone and cyclosporine in the treatment of severe Graves' ophthalmopathy N Engl J Med 1989; 321: 1353-1359.

24. Prummel MF, Mourits MP, Blank L, *et al.* Randomized double-blind trial of prednisone versus radiotherapy in Graves' ophthalmopathy. Lancet 1993; 342: 949-954.

25. Donaldson SS, Bagshaw MA, Kriss JP. Supervoltage orbital radiotherapy for Graves' ophthalmopathy. J Clin Endocrinol Metab 1973; 37: 276-285.

26. Bartalena L, Marcocci C, Chiovato L, *et al.* Orbital Cobalt irradiation combined with systemic corticosteroids for Graves' ophthalmopathy: Comparison with systemic corticosteroids alone. J Clin Endocrinol Metab 1983; 56: 1139-1144.

27. Marcocci C, Bartalena L, Bogazzi F, Bruno-Bossio G, Lepri A, Pinchera A. Orbital radiotherapy combined with high dose systemic glucocorticoids for Graves' ophthalmopathy is more effective than radiotherapy alone: results of a prospective randomized study. J Endocrinol Invest 1991; 14: 853-860.

28. Musch DC, Frueh BR, Landis R. The reliability of Hertel exophthalmometry. Observer variation between physician and lay readers. Ophthalmology 1985; 92: 1177-1180.

29. Van Dijk HJL. Orbital Graves' disease. A modification of the "NO SPECS" classification. Ophthalmology 1981; 88: 479-483.

30. Sergott RC, Felberg NT, Savino PJ, Blizzard JJ, Schatz NJ. Graves' ophthalmopathy - immunologic parameters related to corticosteroid therapy. Invest Ophthalmol Vis Sci 1981; 20: 173-182.

31. Mourits MP, Koornneef L, Wiersinga WM, Prummel MF, Berghout A, Van der Gaag R. Clinical criteria for the assessment of disease activity in Graves' ophthalmopathy: a novel approach. British Journal of Ophthalmology 1989; 73: 639-644.

32. Mourits MP, Prummel MF, Wiersinga WM, Koornneef L. Clinical activity score as a guide in the management of patients with Graves' ophthalmopathy. Clin Endocrinol 1997; 47: 9-14.

33. Rose GE. Commentary. Clinical activity score as a guide in the management of patients with Graves' orbitopathy. Clin Endocrinol 1996; 47: 15

34. Lane C, Feyi-Wabosa A, Lazarus J. A simple scoring system for thyroid eye disease. Abstract book VIth International Symposium on Graves' Ophthalmopathy, Amsterdam 1998; 13(Abstract)

35. Armstrong P, Keevil SF. Magnetic resonance imaging-1: basic principles of image production. Br Med J 1991; 303: 35-40.

36. Just M, Kahaly G, Higer HP, *et al.* Graves' ophthalmopathy: Role of MR Imaging in radiation therapy. Radiology 1991; 179: 187-190.

37. Utech CI, Khatibnia U, Winter PF, Wulle KG. MR T2 relaxation time for the assessment of retrobulbar inflammation in Graves' ophthalmopathy. Thyroid 1995; 5: 185-193.

38. Nakahara H, Noguchi S, Murakami N, *et al*. Graves' ophthalmopathy: MR evaluation of 10-Gy versus 24-Gy irradiation combined with systemic corticosteroids. Radiology 1995; 196: 857-862.

39. Laitt RD, Hoh B, Wakeley C, *et al*. The value of the short tau inversion recovery sequence in magnetic resonance imaging of thyroid eye disease. Br J Radiol 1994; 67: 244-247.

40. Hiromatsu Y, Kojima K, Ishisaka N, *et al*. Role of Magnetic Resonance Imaging in thyroid-associated ophthalmopathy: Its predictive value for therapeutic outcome of immunosuppressive therapy. Thyroid 1992; 2: 299-305.

41. Postema PTE, Krenning EP, Wijngaarde R, *et al*. [111In-DTPA-D-Phe1] octreotide scintigraphy in thyroidal and orbital Graves' disease: a parameter for disease activity? J Clin Endocrinol Metab 1994; 79: 1845-1994.

42. Moncayo R, Baldnisera I, Decristoforo C, Kendler D, Donnemiller E. Evaluation of immunological mechanisms mediating thyroid-associated ophthalmopathy by radionuclide imaging the somatostatin analog ^{111}In-octreotide. Thyroid 1997; 7: 21-29.

43. Kahaly G, Diaz M, Just M, Beyer J, Lieb W. Role of octreoscan and correlation with MR Imaging in Graves' ophthalmopathy. Thyroid 1995; 5: 107-111.

44. Kahaly G, Diaz M, Haka K, Beyer J, Bockisch A. Indium-111-pentetreotide scintigraphy in Graves' ophthalmopathy. J Nucl Med 1995; 36: 550-554.

45. Wiersinga WM, Gerding MN, Prummel MF, Krenning EP. Octreotide scintigraphy in thyroidal and orbital Graves' disease. Thyroid 1998; 8: 433-436.

46. Kahaly G, Gorges R, Diaz M, Hommel G, Bockisch A. Indium-111-Pentetreotide in Graves' disease. J Nucl Med 1998; 39: 533-536.

47. Gerding MN, Van der Zant FM, Van Royen EA, *et al*. Octreotide-scintigraphy is a disease activity parameter in Graves' ophthalmopathy. Clin Endocrinol 1999; 50:373-379.

48. Colao A, Lastoria S, Ferone D, *et al*. Orbital scintigraphy with [111In-Diethylenetriamine Pentaacetic Acid-D-Phe1]-Octreotide predicts the clinical response to corticosteroid therapy in patients with Graves' ophthalmopathy. J Clin Endocrinol Metab 1998; 83: 3790-3794.

49. Krassas GE, Dumas A, Pontikides N, Kaltsas T. Somatostatin receptor scintigraphy and octreotide treatment in patients with thyroid eye disease. Clin Endocrinol 1995; 42: 571-580.

50. Sergott RC, Glaser JS. Graves' ophthalmopathy. A clinical and immunologic review. Surv Ophthalmol 1981; 26: 1-21.

51. Prummel MF, Suttorp-Schulten MS, Wiersinga WM, Verbeek AM, Mourits MP, Koornneef L. A new ultrasonographic method to detect disease activity and predict response to immunosuppressive treatment in Graves ophthalmopathy Ophthalmology 1993; 100: 556-561.

52. Barnes A. Measurement of serum cytokines. Lancet 1998; 352: 324-325.

53. Sergott RC, Felberg NT, Savino PJ, Blizzard JJ, Schatz NJ. E-rosette formation in Graves' ophthalmopathy. Invest Ophthalmol Vis Sci 1979; 18: 1245-1251.

54. Wall JR, Gray B, Greenwood DM. Total and "activated" peripheral blood T lymphocytes in patients with thyroid disorders. Acta Endocrinol (Copenh) 1977; 85: 753-759.

55. Munro RE, Lamki L, Row VV, Volpe R. Cell-mediated immunity in the exophthalmos of Graves' disease as demonstrated by the Migration Inhibition Factor (MIF) test. J Clin Endocrinol Metab 1973; 37: 286-292.

56. Volpe R. Review The role of autoimmunity in hypoendocrine and hyperendocrine function. Ann Int Med 1977; 87: 86-99.

57. Van der Gaag R, Broersma L, Mourits MP, *et al*. Circulating monocyte migration inhibitory factor in serum of Graves' ophthalmopathy patients: a parameter for disease activity? Clin Exp Immunol 1989; 75: 275-279.

58. Balazs C, Farid NR. Soluble Interleukin-2 receptor in sera of patients with Graves' dosease. J Autoimmunity 1991; 4: 681-688.

59. Prummel MF, Wiersinga WM, Van der Gaag R, Mourits MP, Koornneef L. Soluble IL-2 receptor levels in patients with Graves' ophthalmopathy. Clin Exp Immunol 1992; 88: 405-409.

60. Salvi M, Girasole G, Pedrazzoni M, *et al*. Increased serum concentrations of Interleukin-6 (IL-6) and soluble IL-6 Receptor in patients with Graves' disease. J Clin Endocrinol Metab 1996; 81: 2976-2979.

61. Okumura M, Hidaka Y, Kuroda S, Takeoka K, Tada H, Amino N. Increased serum concentration of soluble CD30 in patients with Graves' disease and Hashimoto's thyroiditis. J Clin Endocrinol Metab 1997; 82: 1757-1760.

62. Tan GH, Dutton CM, Bahn RS. Interleukin-1 (IL-1) Receptor Antagonist and soluble IL-1 Receptor inihibit IL-1 induced glycosaminoglycan production in cultured human orbital fibroblasts from patients with Graves' ophthalmopathy. J Clin Endocrinol Metab 1996; 81: 449-452.

63. Hofbauer LC, Muhlberg T, Konig A, Heufelder G, Schworm H, Heufelder AE. Soluble Interleukin-1 receptor antagonist serum levels in smokers and nonsmokers with Graves' ophthalmopathy undergoing orbital radiotherapy. J Clin Endocrinol Metab 1997; 82: 2244-2247.

64. Frenette PS, Wagner DD. Molecular Medicine. Adhesion molecules - Part I. N Engl J Med 1996; 334: 1526-1529.

65. Frenette PS, Wagner DD. Molecular medicine. Adhesion molecules - Part II: blood vessels and blood cells. N Engl J Med 1996; 335: 43-45.

66. Heufelder AE, Bahn RS. Elevated expression *in situ* of selectin and immunoglobulin superfamily type adhesion molecules in retroocular connective tissues from patients with Graves' ophthalmopathy. Clin Exp Immunol 1993; 91: 381-389.

67. Pappa A, Calder V, Fells P, Lightman S. Adhesion molecule expression *in vivo* on extraocular muscles (EOM) in thyroid-associated ophthalmopathy (TAO). Clin Exp Immunol 1997; 108: 3069-313.

68. Heufelder AE, Bahn RS. Soluble intercellular adhesion molecule-1 (sICAM-1) in sera of patients with Graves' ophthalmopathy and thyroid disease. Clin Exp Immunol 1993; 92: 296-302.

69. De Bellis A, Bizzarro A, Gattoni A, *et al*. Behavior of soluble Intercellular Adhesion Molecule-1 and Endothelial-Leukocyte Adhesion molecule-1 concentrations in patients with Graves' disease with or without ophthalmopathy and in patients with toxic adenoma. J Clin Endocrinol Metab 1995; 80: 2118-2121.

70. Prummel MF, Van Pareren Y, Bakker O, Wiersinga WM. Anti-heat shock protein (hsp) 72 antibodies are present in patients with Graves' disease (GD) and in control smoking subjects. Clin Exp Immunol 1997; 110: 292-295.

71. McGregor AM. Has the target autoantigen for Graves' ophthalmopathy been found? Lancet 1998; 352: 595-596.

72. McLachlan SM, Bahn RS, Rapoport B. Endocrine ophthalmopathy: a re-evaluation of the association with thyroid autoantibodies. Autoimmunity 1992; 14: 143-148.

73. Jacobson DH, Gorman CA. Endocrine ophthalmopathy: current ideas concerning etiology, pathogenesis, and treatment. Endocr Rev 1984; 5: 200-220.

74. Pappa A, Jackson P, Stone J, *et al*. An ultrastructural and systemic analysis of glycosaminoglycans in thyroid-associated ophthalmopathy. Eye 1998; 12: 237-244.

75. Smith TJ, Bahn RS, Gorman CA. Connective tissue, glycosaminoglycans, and diseases of the thyroid. Endocr Rev 1989; 10: 366-391.

76. Kahaly G, Schuler M, Sewell AC, Bernhard G, Beyer J, Krause U. Urinary glycosaminoglycans in Graves' ophthalmopathy. Clin Endocrinol 1990; 33: 35-44.

77. Martinez-Bru C, Ampudia X, Castrillo P, Gonzalez-Sastre F. Urinary glycosaminoglycans in active Graves' ophthalmopathy. Clin Chem 1992; 38: 2341

78. Hansen C, Fraiture B, Rouhi R, Otto E, Forster G, Kahaly G. HPLC glycosaminoglycan analysis in patients with Graves' disease. Cli Sci 1997; 92: 511-517.

79. Kahaly G, Forster G, Hansen C. Glycosaminoglycans in Thyroid Eye Disease. Thyroid 1998; 8: 429-432.

80. Kahaly G, Hansen C, Beyer J, Winand R. Plasma glycosaminoglycans in endocrine ophthalmopathy. J Endocrinol Invest 1994; 17: 45-50.

81. Mourits MP, Prummel MF, Wiersinga WM, Koornneef L. Measuring eye movements in Graves' ophthalmopathy. Ophthalmology 1994; 101: 1341-1346.

Chapter 5

Recommendations for the assessment of Therapeutic Outcome of Graves' ophthalmopathy in clinical trials

Aldo Pinchera,* Wilmar M. Wiersinga.
Department of Endocrinology, University of Pisa, Via Paradisa 2, 56124 Pisa, Italy

1.   INTRODUCTION

Graves' ophthalmopathy (GO) is characterized by an array of anatomical changes of the orbital structures. Even though the etiology of GO remains largely unknown, some of the mechanisms leading to these changes and ultimately to the patients' symptoms have been elucidated.[1] Our current understanding of these mechanisms is briefly summarized in Table 1. In the absence of reasonable etiological treatments, these mechanisms are the target of treatments aiming at modifying the natural history of the disease and at preventing its complications. As in many other disorders, in GO there are no measurable metabolic parameters consistently correlating to the severity and activity of the disease and complex anatomical changes need to be measured in order to evaluate the effectiveness of treatments. Different mechanisms may be active in different patients. For example, one patient may have prominent extraocular muscle involvement with marked diplopia without significant proptosis, while the opposite may be true in another patient. How will we compare the severity of the disease in these two patients? Moreover, the disease itself is characterized by a wavelike behavior, with periods of partial spontaneous remission following the initial flare-up, making it difficult to distinguish between the natural history of the disease and the effect of treatments. These problems have represented a major obstacle in the interpretation of the results of clinical trials and their transfer to clinical practice world-wide.

Table 1. Clinical findings in Graves' ophthalmopathy, their pathogenetic mechanisms, and anatomical correlates

Clinical finding	Pathogenetic mechanism	Anatomical correlate
Proptosis	Increased retrobulbar pressure	Swelling of retrobulbar muscle and connective tissue
Visual field defect	Compression of optic nerves	Swelling of retrobulbar muscle and connective tissue
Diplopia	Impaired extraocular muscle contraction	Shortening and infiltration of extraocular muscle
Corneal ulceration and exposure keratitits	Proptosis and/or impaired extraocular muscle contraction	Swelling of retrobulbar muscle and connective tissue; shortening and infiltration of elevator muscles
Palpebral edema, chemosis, conjunctival inflammation	Venous stasis	Swelling of retrobulbar muscle and connective tissue

2.   CURRENT CONCEPTS

Initial studies taking into account only variations in one parameter (proptosis) have been superseded by the introduction of the Ophthalmopathy Index (OI), by Donaldson,[2] which represents a refinement of the classification originally proposed by Werner. This scoring method is based on the summation of individual semi-quantitative scores obtained at one of the possible "points of involvement" of GO (NOSPECS classification), which included: moderate signs only, no symptoms (O) soft tissue (S), proptosis (P), extraocular muscle (E), corneal involvement (C), optic nerve (S). Although this score has represented a first effort to give the scientific community a standardized tool for measuring eye-changes related to GO, it has raised some criticism. First, in its original formulation, the numerical value given to each of the six parameters derives basically from the subjective evaluation of the observer, making the measurements difficult to reproduce. Second, the index derives from the summation of scores on different parameters that are often independent of each other. Therefore, changes in the score may not adequately reflect real changes in the severity of the disease. For example, a patient whose proptosis score is decreased from 3 to 1 following surgical decompression, but whose diplopia score increases from 0 to 2, would have a total score that is unchanged, but it would be hard to claim that this patient's ophthalmopathy has not changed in response to treatment! Third, it has been suggested that the NOSPECS classification takes into account findings that are indirect and late consequences of the disease.[3] Following this view, an effort should be made to measure events that are closer to the primum movens of the clinical manifestations of the disease, in order to obtain more specific data. The NOSPECS classification remains a useful mnemonic tool for educational and also for clinical purposes. The ophthalmopathy index (O.I.) derived from the NOSPECS classification may not be appropriate as the sole method for reporting original data on experimental treatments for GO. In this view, in 1992 an ad hoc Committee of the Four Sister Thyroid Societies reviewed the problem of the classification of eye changes in GO and proposed that only the objective measurements listed in Table 2 should be used in reporting clinical trials of treatment of GO.[4] However, the committee also stated that the inclusion of some subjective features (Clinical Activity Score, CAS), as well as the patients' perception of their disease activity is of great value in fully evaluating the severity of the disease.[5] The Committee recommended a reevaluation of the above criteria after five years.

Table 2. Measurements recommended by the Sister Societies *ad hoc* Committee for the Classification of eye changes in Graves' ophthalmopathy (1992).[5]

Orbital structure	Measurement
Eye lids	Maximum lid fissure
Cornea	Presence or absence of exposure keratitits
Extraocular muscle	Presence or absence of single binocular vision in the central 30° of visual fields.
	Maddox rod test, alternate cover test, Hess chart, or Lancaster red-green test.
	Volume measurement by CT, ultrasound or MRI, or cross-sectional diameter measurement of extraocular muscle.
Retrobulbar tissue as a whole	Exophthalmometer readings
Optic nerve	Visual acuity, visual fields, or color vision

3.   RECOMMENDATIONS FOR CLINICAL TRIALS ADDRESSING THE TREATMENT OF GO

3.1   Study Design

Clinicians and scientists designing new studies of GO treatment should always follow the general principles of evidence-based medicine. Therefore, only carefully controlled, prospective, randomized studies can be considered acceptable. Placebo treated controls are always desirable and represent a very efficient way to correct for changes in disease severity that may be ascribed to natural history alone. However, placebo controlled studies may not always be feasible because of ethical considerations. Therefore control groups treated with alternative or established treatment protocols are suitable, provided they are correctly randomized.

3.2   Characterization of patients

Even though sound randomization should correct for confounding factors, it is recommended that factors already known to interfere with the disease history should be carefully sought and described in patients. Only few risk factors are known to modulate the clinical expression of GO. These include age, sex and family history. Tobacco smoke has recently emerged as a major risk factor for both the presence and severity of GO in GD patients and should therefore always reported.[1] Radioiodine treatment of thyrotoxicosis is also a factor (see below). Data on these factors should be sought and reported in all series.

Optimally, only patients without history of previous treatments for GO should be included. When this is not possible, for example when second step treatments are being evaluated, history of previous treatments should be collected and reported in detail.

3.3   Treatment of thyroid dysfunction

The treatment of thyroid dysfunction is also thought to have an impact on the course of GO. Transient worsening of GO has been observed after radioiodine treatment for hyperthyroidism.[6,7] The timing of radioiodine administration with respect to the treatment for GO being studied should therefore be carefully reported and should not differ between cases and controls. When definitive treatment of thyrotoxicosis is being performed before treatment of GO, all patients in the study should be stably euthyroid on l-T4 therapy at the time of initiation of the protocol. This should be documented by TSH and thyroid hormone measurements. When the study protocol does not include preliminary definitive treatment of thyrotoxicosis by either thyroidectomy or radioiodine, thyroid function at baseline should not be different between different groups of patients and patients should be maintained euthyroid by anti-thyroid drug therapy throughout the study.

3.4   Measures of changes upon treatment

Since the release of the recommendations of the ad hoc committee in 1992, a number of studies on the treatment of GO have been published in international journals. The choice among the many available measures should be tailored on the aims of the treatment being studied. As stated above, a single index of ophthalmopathy obtained from the summation of scores at different end-points may be misleading and should not be used as the only assessment of the effects of treatment. It appears therefore very important that investigators report in clinical trials effects on single manifestations of GO, in the view that some treatments may be more active on some manifestations of the disease.

3.4.1   Proptosis

Measurement of proptosis may be efficiently obtained by Hertel exophthalmometer readings. Although normal values may vary in different ethnic groups,[8] changes in proptosis of more than 2 mm in a single individual are significant and reproducible. Repeat CT and MRI scan measures of proptosis are also acceptable for clinical studies.

3.4.2   Extraocular muscle dysfunction

Changes in ocular motility can be reliably quantitated by a number of methods, such as the Maddox rod test, the Hess chart, the Lancaster red-green test and others.[3] Other methods using modified perimeters have been specifically validated for use in GO, and can be used as well.

3.4.3   Lid aperture

Lid fissure measurement with a simple ruler is an indirect measure of both levator muscle dysfunction and measurement. The method has not been rigorously validated. The distance between the lower and the upper lid should be taken with the patient at rest, looking straight ahead. The measurement should always be performed in the morning, in order to avoid changes due to circadian variations in the sympathetic tone.

3.4.4   Measures of orbital tissues

Since the major single pathogenetic event in GO is an increase in the volume of orbital tissues, efforts should be made to provide a reliable and reproducible measure of this entity. Measurements of muscle size based on cross-sectional diameter obtained with either CT, MRI or ultrasound is imprecise due to the wide effect of small differences in the angle at which the section is acquired at different times. Therefore, direct, computer-assisted CT scan analysis of the volume of extraocular muscles and orbital fat should be employed when reporting treatments expected to affect this aspect.[9]

3.4.5   Optic nerve dysfunction

Quantitative measurements of optic nerve dysfunction should be reported by standard studies of visual acuity, visual fields and color vision. More sophisticated techniques, such as evoked visual potential and others are not required but may be provided.

3.4.6   Corneal involvement

Objective quantitation of progression or partial regression of pre-existing exposure keratitis is difficult to obtain, only the emergence of new corneal lesions or the disappearance of pre-existing ones during or after the proposed treatment should be taken into account.

3.4.7   Activity of GO

It has been suggested that inflammatory phenomena predominate during the early phases of the disease, determining many aspects of its clinical presentation, including a number of clinical signs that can be evaluated during examination of patients. According to this view, accurate determination of inflammatory signs such as pain, chemosis, palpebral edema, conjunctival injection, edema of the caruncula and others may be of help in evaluating the effect of early immune suppressive treatment. Other signs, that may be present also in long standing, "inactive" ophthalmopathy, such as proptosis, eye muscle or optic nerve dysfunction have been included as markers of active inflammation when changing over a short period of time. Based on these signs, a numeric clinical activity score (CAS)[5] has been proposed. Although the CAS has been validated in clinical studies and shown to efficiently identify patients more likely to respond to immune suppression, it still relies on qualitative or at best semiquantitative subjective parameters. Moreover, the link between the inflammatory process and the parameters included in the CAS is weak. For example, conjunctival injection may be a consequence of locally released cytokines during active inflammation, as well as of long standing impaired orbital venous drainage. In spite of these problems, however, the CAS still represents the best available tool for the description of the elusive concept of activity of GO, and should be used when short term effects of immune suppressive treatment are being studied.

4. CONCLUSIONS

Parallel to our incomplete knowledge of the pathogenesis of GO, our tools in the clinical evaluation of patients are far from perfect. However, some objective ways for measuring the effect of treatment of GO are available. These methods should be adopted by investigators uniformly so that results of different treatments can be compared. At the same time it is important to stress the need for more efficient, quantitative methods.

5. REFERENCES

1. Burch HB, Wartofsky L. Graves' ophthalmopathy: Current concepts regarding pathogenesis and management. Endocr Rev 1993;14:747-793.
2. Donaldson SS, Bagshaw MA, Kriss JP. Supervoltage orbital radiotherapy for Graves' ophthalmopathy. J Clin Endocrinol Metab 1973;37:276-285.
3. Gorman CA. The measurement of change in Graves' ophthalmopathy. Thyroid 1998; 8:539-543.
4. Classification of eye changes of Graves' disease. Thyroid 1992; 2:235-236.
5. Mourits MP, Prummel MF, Wiersinga WM, Koornneef L. Clinical activity score as a guide in the management of patients with Graves' ophthalmopathy. Clin Endocrinol 1997; 47:9-14.
6. Bartalena L, Marcocci C, Bogazzi F, *et al.* Relation between therapy for hyperthyroidism and the course of Graves' ophthalmopathy. N Engl J Med 1998; 338:73-78.
7. Hamilton RD, Mayberry WE, McConahey WM, Hanson KC. Ophthalmopathy of Graves' disease: a comparison between patients treated surgically and patients treated with radioiodide. Mayo Clin Proc 1967; 42:812-818.
8. Migliori ME, Gladstone GJ. Determination of the normal range of exophthalmometric value for black and white adults. Am J Ophthalmol 1984; 98:438-442.
9. Forbes G, Gorman CA, Brennan MD, Gehring DG, Ilstrup DM, Earnest Ft. Ophthalmopathy of Graves' disease: computerized volume measurements of the orbital fat and muscle. AJNR 1986; 7:651-656.

Chapter 6

Thyroid management in Graves' ophthalmopathy

Mark F. Prummel,* Wilmar M. Wiersinga, Claudio Marcocci, Anthony P. Weetman

*Department of Endocrinology, F5-171, Academic Medical Center, University of Amsterdam, Meibergdreef 9, 1105 AZ, Amsterdam, The Netherlands

There is a close temporal relationship between the occurrence of Graves' thyroid disease (GTD) and the onset of Graves' ophthalmopathy (Fig. 1).[1] Both Gorman *et al.*, and Wiersinga *et al*, found that in approximately ¾ of the patients both manifestations occurred within 18 months of eachother.[2,3] In the majority, the eye signs develop after the first signs of hyperthyroidism. Although clinically manifest ophthalmopathy is seen in only appr. 35% of the patients with Graves' hyperthyroidism, subclinical evidence for orbital disease is present in almost all patients.[1] This close association has always been the most pertinent reason to think that the ophthalmopathy and the thyroid disorder are actually two manifestations of the same condition: Graves' disease.

However, the temporal association has also fueled the idea that the management of the thyroid disease might affect on the severity and course of the ophthalmopathy. Here we will review the evidence for this hypothesis. First we will focus on the possible effects of thyroid dysfunction itself on the eye disease, and secondly on the question whether the type of thyroid treatment makes a difference for the course of the ophthalmopathy.

1. DOES THYROID FUNCTION AFFECT THE EYES?

It has been the feeling of many authors that an abnormal thyroid function *per se* has an influence on the signs and symptoms of the eye disease.[1] However, this is difficult to prove because the antithyroid drugs used to treat the hyperthyroidism themselves might have an influence on the immune system. It is thus difficult to establish whether a beneficial effect on the eye signs upon reaching euthyroidism is caused by the antithyroid drugs, or by rendering the patient euthyroid. Despite these difficulties, there is evidence that hyperthyroxinemia itself has an effect on the immune system.[4,5] Hyperthyroidism is associated with a decrease in the functional activity of the T suppressor cells.[6] Furthermore, thyrotoxicosis due to exogenous thyroxine administration or toxic nodular goiter induces a decrease in the NK cell activity (cells which control autoantibody production by B lymphocytes).[4,7] On the other hand, hypothyroidism might also have an effect because TSH increases HLA-DR expression on thyrocytes *in vitro*, which might enhance the immune response.[8] Indeed, when patients with Hashimoto's hypothyroidism are treated with thyroxine a decrease in the levels of autoantibodies against TPO and the TSH-Receptor is seen.[9]

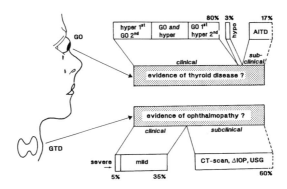

Figure 1. Schematic representation of the evidence for thyroid disease in ophthalmopathy patients (GO), and for eye disease in Graves' thyroid disease (GTD) patients. AITD, autoimmune thyroid disease; Hypo, primary hypothyroidism; USG, ultrasonography; IOP, intraocular pressure. (Contributed by M.F. Prummel)

Thyroid dysfunction might also have an effect directly on the orbital tissues, because β_1 Thyroid Hormone Receptors are abundant in the orbital layers of these muscles.[10] On the other hand there is increasing evidence for the presence of the TSH-Receptor in the orbit, most likely on the orbital fibroblasts (see Chapter 2), and thus in theory elevated TSH levels in hypothyroidism might have an effect directly on these fibroblasts.

Thus, hyper- and hypothyroidism might very well have an effect on the eye disease, both directly or indirectly by influencing the immune system. However, there is only limited clinical evidence for this being the case. One of the few studies addressing this issue was a retrospective study in 90 patients with ophthalmopathy upon referral to an orbital clinic. Fifty-four of them were euthyroid, 36 had either hyper- or hypothyroidism despite antithyroid treatment. The patients were assigned to four different groups with increasing severity of their ophthalmopathy, and it appeared that most of the dysthyroid patients could be found in the more severe ophthalmopathy groups.[11] Also, the dysthyroid patients had more proptosis and a higher overall total eye score. In a second study the eye changes improved significantly in the dysthyroid patients when they were made euthyroid, whereas the ophthalmopathy remained unchanged in the euthyroid patients during a similar follow-up of 20 weeks.[12] These observations thus support the idea that an abnormal thyroid function indeed is associated with more severe ophthalmopathy and that controlling the thyroid function can be beneficial in ophthalmopathy patients.

2. EFFECT OF ANTITHYROID TREATMENT ON THE EYES: IMMUNOLOGICAL MECHANISMS

There is no consensus on the type of antithyroid treatment to be given to a patient with clinically apparent eye disease. In a survey from the European Thyroid Association, experienced thyroidologists were confronted with a female patient with severe ophthalmopathy and asked how they would manage the thyroid disorder.[13] Eighty-four percent of 82 respondents would use antithyroid drugs initially, 10% would perform surgery, and 6% would prefer [131]Iodine treatment. If the patient would have been seen after a recurrence of hyperthyroidism, 43% would now prefer surgery, 25% would give [131]I (often with steroids), and only 32% would use another course of antithyroid drugs. There were wide geographic differences: In The Netherlands the great majority would only use antithyroid drugs, whereas in Germany 31% would perform (near) total thyroidectomy with prophylactic steroids. Which are the reasons to believe that the type of antithyroid therapy might influence the ophthalmopathy?

2.1 Antithyroid drugs

It was noted that the levels of microsomal antibodies, and of TSH-R antibodies decreased in patients treated with carbimazole, as opposed to placebo- or propranolol treated patients, a decrease which was not related to T4 levels.[14] It seems unlikely that this decrease in antibody titers was due to restoration of the euthyroid state itself, because a similar decline in microsomal antibody levels was seen in patients with Hashimoto's disease treated with thyroxine *and* carbimazole.[15] Methimazole was shown to inhibit free oxygen radical formation by monocytes,[16] indirectly decrease the expression of HLA-DR on thyrocytes by lectin,[17] and induce a fall in peripheral T-helper lymphocytes with an increase in T-suppressor cells.[7] These changes are accompanied by a gradual decline in TSH-R antibody levels during therapy with carbimazole.[14,18]

Thus, it appears that antithyroid drugs, though they are not strong immunosuppressive agents, do have some local immunosuppressive effect in the thyroid gland itself, leading to a decrease in antibody levels T-helper/T-suppressor cell ratio.[4,19]

2.2   Radioactive iodine

[131]I is the preferred method to control thyrotoxicosis in many centers, especially in the U.S.A.[20] By itself, the minute amounts of iodine administered will probably not affect the immune system, although the radioactivity might locally affect the intrathyroidal lymphocytes. However, the most likely effect of ^{131}I is through the destruction of thyroid tissue and the subsequent liberation of thyroidal antigens which will be presented to the immune system.[21] This exposure might stimulate the autoantibody production against thyroidal antigens, including the putative antibodies crossreacting with an orbital antigen. A candidate for this is the TSH-Receptor, and indeed many studies have shown that the levels of TSH-R antibodies increase substantially in the months after administration of radioactive iodine.[22,23] The clinical relevance of this increase in TSH-R antibody levels 3-6 months after ^{131}I has recently been recognized in a completely different setting. Graves-like hyperthyroidism is a side effect of ^{131}I treatment of large multinodular goiters, occurring in 4% of the patients after 3-6 months in conjunction with the *de novo* appearance of TSH-R antibodies.[24,25] Radioactive iodine also affects the cellular immune response against the TSH-Receptor, and more in general ^{131}I treatment is followed by an increase in T cell reactivity.[26,27]

2.3   Thyroid surgery

The slow destruction of thyroid tissues by radioactive iodine and the release of antigens thus stimulates the production of antithyroidal autoantibodies. By the same token, removal of all thyroid tissue and thyroidal antigens, might down regulate the immune system and lead to a decrease in thyroidal antibody levels. Bauer and Catz therefore advocated *total* thyroid ablation, which can be reached by either surgery or radioactive iodine (or both), and reported that this treatment resulted in a complete regression of the eye changes in 32 patients.[28] These findings could not be confirmed by Werner *et al.*, but in their study not all thyroid tissue could be removed and thus the aforementioned hypothesis was not vitiated.[29] Marcocci *et al.* reviewed a number of uncontrolled studies and came to the conclusion that a lack of beneficial effect on the orbital disease after total thyroidectomy could be attributed to the fact that residual thyroid tissue was usually still present after the procedure.[5] Thus, although the original idea may not have been repudiated, there is no sound evidence for the claimed beneficial effect. Nevertheless, it appears to be an attractive hypothesis, for DeGroot uses total thyroid ablation with radioactive iodine to treat his patients with severe ophthalmopathy.[21,30]

Subtotal thyroidectomy is, however, an effective treatment for Graves' hyperthyroidism, and does not seem to lead to a significant increase in the levels of antibodies against TPO and the TSH-Receptor in the months following the procedure.[31] Surgery therefore does not seem to alter the immune reponse, at least not in the long term.

In conclusion, the three treatment modalities have a different effect on the immune system and there is sufficient theoretical basis to assume that they thus might have a different effect on the eye changes in Graves' disease. Now we will review the clinical evidence for the possible different effects on the ophthalmopathy.

3.   EFFECT OF ANTITHYROID TREATMENT ON THE EYES : CLINICAL TRIALS

This subject has been a matter of debate and studies during many decades, which has resulted in a vast literature, which is reviewed excellently elsewhere.[1] As discussed in Chapter 4, the natural course of the ophthalmopathy is characterized by a tendency towards spontaneous improvement. This fact dictates that the results of uncontrolled studies are of very limited value, and therefore we will only comment on the controlled studies. Bahn and Gorman have set important rules for a study that evaluates the effect of a certain treatment on the eye changes.[32] We will use these rules (Table 1) to analyze the various controlled studies published.

One of the first controlled follow-up studies was done by Sridama and DeGroot.[33] They retrospectively reviewed the large number of 426 patients with Graves' thyroid disease of whom 164 were treated surgically, 182 with antithyroid drugs, and 241 by [131]I (80 patients received more than one treatment modality). These treatments were complicated by newly occurring ophthalmopathy in resp 7.1%, 6.7%, and 4.9%, and by progression of preexisting eye disease in 19.2%, 19.8%, 12.3% respectively. These rates were not significantly different and the authors concluded that the choice of antithyroid therapy does not influence the development or exacerbation of the ophthalmopathy. This study has been cited extensively, but can be criticized when applying the rules from Table 1.

Table 1. Suggestions for the optimal interpretation of treatment results in Graves' ophthalmopathy according to Bahn and Gorman.[32]

	Suggestions
1.	Use objective criteria to assess the eye status
2.	Controlled studies should be done whenever possible
3.	During the period of observation, only a single form of treatment should be employed
4.	The interval between therapy and assessment of results should be sufficiently short to make spontaneous improvement or worsening unlikely. Three months is probably optimal, with 6 months being the maximum allowable interval.
5.	Each patient should be euthyroid throughout the period of observation

Firstly, the study was not properly controlled and the patients differed in various important base-line characteristics (age, sex, thyroid hormone levels), and patients with severe eye disease were not subjected to radioactive iodine. Secondly, in 80/426 patients (19%) more than a single therapy was given. Thirdly, and most importantly, the mean interval between treatment and assessment of result was 5.0 ± 3.2 years (range: 1-11 years). After such a long follow-up the eye disease will have stabilized in many patients at a certain level of severity (see Rundle's curve), and the short term effects of the antithyroid therapy on the eye disease was thus not assessed at the recommended 3-6 months. Lastly, 54% of the patients from the surgical group, and 29% of the ^{131}I group had previously been treated with antithyroid drugs elsewhere, in contrast to only 9% in the medically treated patient group. Thus, the antithyroid drug treated patients had a shorter duration of their Graves' disease and thus had a higher probability for deterioration of the eye disease. In summary, the study largely reported the natural history of these patients, and no conclusions on the differential effect of the applied therapies on the ophthalmopathy are warranted.

After this report several truly randomized trials have been performed. The first compared the occurrence of ophthalmopathy among patients treated with antithyroid drugs, radioactive iodine, and subtotal thyroidectomy.[34] This study was slightly complicated because the authors did not want to use ^{131}I therapy in younger patients, and the 54 patients between 20 and 34 years of age were randomized to surgery or to antithyroid drug treatment (Methimazole 4 dd. 10 mg), with thyroxine substitution in both arms to prevent hypothyroidism. The outcome regarding the ophthalmopathy was assessed at monthly intervals for one year. The outcome was similar in both treatment arms: worsening of preexisting eye disease, or new development of ophthalmopathy occurred in 15% in the medical group, and in 11% in the surgical group. The 114 older patients (35-55 yrs old) were randomized to receive antithyroid drug therapy (n=38), radioactive iodine (n=39), or subtotal thyroidectomy (n=37). The randomization was successful since the baseline characteristics were similar in the three groups. In this age group there was significant difference in outcome of the eye disease. New development or exacerbation of ophthalmopathy occurred in 10% of the drug treated patients, in 16% of the surgically treated patients, but in 33% of the ^{131}I treated patients (P=0.02). The risk for the eyes was also higher when pretreatment T_3 levels were higher (Fig. 2). Although this was a truly randomized and prospective study, it was criticized quite heavily.[1,35] The most important criticism being that in the ^{131}I group the patients were allowed to develop hypothyroidism before thyroxine substitution was administered, whereas in the other two groups thyroxine was given prophylactically. This was indeed a violation of rule 5 of Table 1, and raised TSH levels are indeed associated with more severe ophthalmopathy (see above). However, in a retrospective analysis, TSH levels did not determine whether a ^{131}I treated patient had worsening or new developed ophthalmopathy, and prophylactic T_4 administration right after radioiodine did only partially protect against this event.[36]

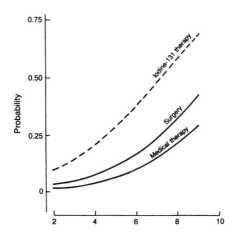

Figure 2. Probability of the development or worsening of ophthalmopathy in patients with Graves' hyperthyroidism. (Reproduced with permission from the Publisher.[34])

Earlier Bartalena *et al* showed that worsening of ophthalmopathy after radioiodine could be prevented with a 3 month course of corticosteroids.[37] In this study ophthalmopathy developed or worsened in 56% of patients treated with ^{131}I alone, an event which did not occur in the patients randomized to ^{131}I and a 3 month course of corticosteroids. Unfortunately, no control group treated with another antithyroid therapy (like antithyroid drugs) was included in this study. This omission did not occur in another randomized clinical trial by the same group from Pisa.[38] Here 443 patients with no or slight ophthalmopathy were randomized to receive radioiodine (n=150), radioiodine and prednisone (n=145), or methimazole only (n=148). In this study baseline characteristics were similar among the groups (including the number of smokers), and hypo- or hyperthyroidism was promptly corrected. The patients were followed at 1-2 month intervals for one year, with emphasis on the eye status. The results are presented in Table 2.

Table 2. Development of Graves' ophthalmopathy (GO), or worsening of pre-existing eye disease in patients with Graves' hyperthyroidism treated with two different antithyroid therapy modalities (Bartalena *et al.*[38])

	Radioiodine	Radioiodine	Methimazole	Methimazole
	No GO	GO present	No GO	GO present
Number of patients / group	78	72	74	74
No change	72	55	72	68
Improvement	-	0	-	3
Development or worsening	6	17	1	3
GO needing treatment	1	7	0	1

   In summary, especially in patients with pre-existing ophthalmopathy there was a true, though small risk for worsening of the eye changes after therapy with radioactive iodine (P<0.001). Whereas antithyroid drug treatment was associated with improvement in 3/78 (4%) of patients with preexisting ophthalmopathy and with an equal number of 3/78 (4%) patients who had progression of the eye disease, none of the radioiodine treated patients improved, and 17/72 (24%) with preexisting ophthalmopathy worsened. Seven of the 72 patients with pre-existing ophthalmopathy (10%) in the radioiodine group needed immunosuppressive therapy, in contrast to only 1/78 (1%) in the methimazole group.

   Thus, the two prospective studies reached the same conclusion that ^{131}I therapy carries a small, but not negligible risk to aggravate pre-existing ophthalmopathy. Whether this is causally related to the radioiodine therapy, or whether antithyroid drugs have a prophylactic effect remains unclear.[39] The risk for new ophthalmopathy to develop upon ^{131}I treatment is low, and probably negligible.[40]

The third treatment option is thyroidectomy. There are no controlled studies involving total thyroid ablation (see above), and whether subtotal thyroidectomy has any effect on the eye disease is uncertain. Reviewing the uncontrolled studies, there is little clinical evidence that surgery has a deleterious effect on the eyes.[1,5] In the prospective, randomized study mentioned no significant difference regarding the outcome of the ophthalmopathy was found between methimazole therapy and subtotal thyroidectomy in the younger age group.[34] During the VIth International Symposium, Marcocci demonstrated that subtotal thyroidectomy was followed by worsening of ophthalmopathy in only a small minority (2/30, 7%) of prospectively followed patients.[41]

4. CONCLUSIONS AND RECOMMENDATIONS

Although the thyroid disease and the ophthalmopathy can run different courses, there is now sufficient evidence that the treatment of the thyroid disease can have an effect on the eye changes. It seems reasonable to state that in a patient with Graves' ophthalmopathy a meticulous control of thyroid function is an important first step in the treatment of the eye disease. The best way to achieve this euthyroidism has been a matter of debate over the last decades. From this debate, finally a number of prospective, controlled trials has emerged with essentially the same conclusions: radioactive iodine carries a higher risk for an exacerbation of pre-existing ophthalmopathy, in comparison to thyroidectomy and antithyroid drug treatment.

On the basis of the available evidence it seems therefore that antithyroid drugs are the treatment of choice to control hyperthyroidism in a patient presenting with ophthalmopathy. There is an approximate 50% risk for recurrent Graves' hyperthyroidism after a course of methimazole and in this case a definitive treatment will be suggested. From the above mentioned studies it is probably safe (for the eyes) to perform a thyroidectomy in such a patient. A second option, also based on evidence, is radioactive iodine with a 3-month course of corticosteroids to prevent an exacerbation of the eye changes. In the Orbital Center in Amsterdam, a third strategy is followed consisting of continuation of the antithyroid drugs until the ophthalmopathy has completely been inactivated and the patient's eye condition is rehabilitated surgically. Thus, they frequently receive methimazole with thyroxine for 2-5 years.

5.   REFERENCES

1. Burch H, Wartofsky L. Graves' ophthalmopathy: Current concepts regarding pathogenesis and management. Endocr Rev 1993; 14: 747-793.
2. Gorman CA. Temporal relationship between onset of Graves' ophthalmopathy and diagnosis of thyrotoxicosis. Mayo Clin Proc 1983; 58: 515-519.
3. Wiersinga WM, Smit T, Van der Gaag R, Koornneef L. Temporal relationship between onset of Graves' ophthalmopathy and onset of thyroidal Graves' disease. J Endocrinol Invest 1988; 11: 615-619.
4. Volpe R. Evidence that the immunosuppressive effects of antithyroid drugs are mediated through actions on the thyroid cell, modulating thyrocyte-immunocyte signalling: a review. Thyroid 1994; 2: 217-223.
5. Marcocci C, Bartalena L, Bogazzi F, Bruno-Bossio G, Pinchera A. Relationship between Graves' ophthalmopathy and type of treatment of Graves' hyperthyroidism. Thyroid 1992; 2: 171-178.
6. Volpe R. Immunoregulation in autoimmune thyroid disease. N Engl J Med 1987; 316: 44-46.
7. Papic M, Stein-Streilein J, Zakarija M, McKenzie JM, Guffee J, Fletcher MA. Suppression of peripheral blood Natural Killer cell activity by excess thyroid hormone. J Clin Invest 1987; 79: 404-408.
8. Todd I, Pujol-Borrel R, Hammond LJ, Nally JM, Feldmann M, Botazzo GF. Enhancement of thyrocyte HLA class II expresion by thyroid-stimulating hormone. Clin Exp Immunol 1987; 69: 524-531.
9. Rieu M, Richard A, Rosilio M, *et al.* Effects of thyroid status on thyroid autoimmunity expression in euthyroid and hypothyroid patients with Hashimoto's thyroiditis. Clin Endocrinol 1994; 40: 529-535.
10. Schmidt ED, Schmidt EDL, Van der Gaag R, *et al.* Distribution of the nuclear thyroid-hormone receptor in extraocular and skeletal muscles. J Endocrinol 1992; 133: 67-74.
11. Prummel MF, Wiersinga WM, Mourits MP, Koornneef L, Berghout A, Van der Gaag R. Effect of abnormal thyroid function on the severity of Graves' ophthalmopathy. Arch Int Med 1990; 150: 1098-1101.
12. Prummel MF, Wiersinga WM, Mourits MP, Koornneef L, Berghout A, Van der Gaag R. Amelioration of eye changes of Graves' ophthalmopathy by achieving euthyroidism. Acta Endocrinol (Copenh) 1989; 121(Suppl.2): 185-189.
13. Weetman AP, Wiersinga WM. Current management of thyroid-associated ophthalmopathy in Europe. Results of an international survey. Clin Endocrinol 1998; 49: 21-28.
14. McGregor AM, Petersen MM, McLachlan SM, Rooke P, Smith BR, Hall R. Carbimazole and the autoimmune response in Graves' disease. N Engl J Med 1980; 303: 302-307.
15. McGregor AM, Ibbertson HK, Rees Smith B, Hall R. Carbimazole and autoantibody synthesis in Hashimoto's thyroiditis. Br Med J 1980; 281: 968-969.
16. Weetman AP, Holt ME, Campbell AK, Hall R, McGregor AM. Methimazole and generation of oxygen radicals by monocytes: potential role in immunosuppression. Br Med J 1984; 288: 518-520.
17. Davies TF, Yang C, Platzer M. The influence of antithyroid drugs and iodine on thyroid cell MHC class II antigen presentation. Clin Endocrinol 1989; 31: 125-135.
18. Pinchera A, Liberti P, Martino E, *et al.* Effects of antithyroid drug therapy on the long acting thyroid stimulator and antithyroglobulin antibodies. J Clin Endocrinol Metab 1969; 29: 231-238.

19. Weetman AP. The immunomodulatory effects of antithyroid drugs. Thyroid 1994; 2: 145-146.
20. Soloman B, Glinoer D, Lagasse R, Wartofsky L. Current trends in the management of Graves' disease. J Clin Endocrinol Metab 1990; 70: 1518-1524.
21. DeGroot LJ. Radioiodine and the immune system. Thyroid 1997; 7: 259-264.
22. McGregor AM, Petersen MM, Capiferri R, Evered DC, Smith BR, Hall R. Effects of radioiodine on thyrotropin binding inhibiting immunoglobulins in Graves' disease. Clin Endocrinol 1979; 11: 437-444.
23. Pinchera A, Pinchera MG, Stanbury JB. Thyrotropin and long acting thyroid stimulator assays in thyroid disease. J Clin Endocrinol Metab 1965; 25: 189-208.
24. Nygaard B, Hegedus L, Gervil M, Hjalgrim H, Soe-Jensen P, Hansen JM. Radioiodine treatment of multinodular non-toxic goitre. Br Med J 1993; 307: 828-832.
25. Huysmans DAKC, Hermus ARMM, Edelbroek MAL, *et al.* Autoimmune hyperthyroidism occurring late after radioiodine treatment for volume reduction of large multinodular goiters. Thyroid 1997; 7: 535-539.
26. Teng WP, Stark R, Munro AJ, Young SM, Borysewicz LK, Weetman AP. Peripheral blood T cell activation after radioiodine treatment for Graves' disease. Acta Endocrinol (Copenh) 1990; 122: 233-240.
27. Soliman M, Kaplan E, Abdel-Latif A, Scherberg N, DeGroot LJ. Does thyroidectomy, radioactive iodine therapy, or antithyroid drug treatment alter reactivity of patients' T cells to epitopes of thyrotropin receptor in autoimmune thyroid diseases? J Clin Endocrinol Metab 1995; 80: 2312-2321.
28. Bauer FK, Catz B. Radioactive iodine therapy for progressive malignant exophthalmos. Acta Endocrinol (Copenh) 1966; 51: 15-22.
29. Werner SC, Feind CR, Aida M. Graves' disease and total thyroidectomy. Progression of severe eye changes and decrease in serum Long Acting Thyroid Stimulator after operation. N Engl J Med 1967; 276: 132-137.
30. DeGroot LJ. Retro-orbital radiation and radioactive iodide ablation of the thyroid may be good for Graves' ophthalmopathy. J Clin Endocrinol Metab 1995; 80: 339-340.
31. De Bruin TWA, Patwardhan A, Brown RS, Braverman LE. Graves' disease: changes in TSH receptor and anti-microsomal antibodies after thyroidectomy. Clin Exp Immunol 1988; 72: 481-485.
32. Bahn RS, Gorman CA. Choice of therapy and criteria for assessing treatment outcome in thyroid-associated ophthalmopathy. Endocrinol Metab Clin North Am 1987; 16: 391-407.
33. Sridama V, DeGroot LJ. Treatment of Graves' disease and the course of ophthalmopathy. AmJ Med 1989; 87: 70-73.
34. Tallstedt L, Lundell G, Torring O, *et al.* Occurrence of ophthalmopathy after treatment for Graves' hyperthyroidism. N Engl J Med 1992; 326: 1733-1738.
35. Gorman CA. Radioiodine therapy does not aggravate Graves' ophthalmopathy. J Clin Endocrinol Metab 1995; 80: 340-342.
36. Tallstedt L, Lundell G, Blomgren H, Bring J. Does early administration of thyroxine reduce the development of Graves' ophthalmopathy after radioiodine treatment? Eur J Endocrinol 1994; 130: 494-497.
37. Bartalena L, Marcocci C, Bogazzi F, Panicucci M, Lepri A, Pinchera A. Use of corticosteroids to prevent progression of Graves' ophthalmopathy after radioiodine therapy for hyperthyroidism. N Engl J Med 1989; 321: 1349-1362.
38. Bartalena L, Marcocci C, Bogazzi F, *et al.* Relation between therapy for hyperthyroidism and the course of Graves' ophthalmopathy. N Engl J Med 1998; 338: 73-78.
39. Wiersinga WM. Preventing Graves' ophthalmopathy. N Engl J Med 1998; 338: 121-122.

40. Barth A, Probst P, Burgi H. Identification of a subgroup of Graves' disease patients at higher risk for severe ophthalmopathy after radioiodine. J Endocrinol Invest 1991; 14: 209-212.
41. Marcocci C, Bartalena L, Pinchera A. Ablative or non-ablative therapy for Graves' hyperthyroidism in patients with ophthalmopathy? J Endocrinol Invest 1998; 21: 468-471.

Chapter 7

Immunosuppressive management of Graves' ophthalmopathy

Claudio Marcocci,* Aldo Pinchera, Mark F. Prummel, Wilmar M. Wiersinga.
*Dept of Endocrinology, University of Pisa, Via Paradisa 2, 56124 Pisa, Italy

Several lines of evidence indicate that Graves' ophthalmopathy (GO) is an autoimmune disorder.[1] Humoral and cell-mediated immune reactions have been implicated in the pathogenesis of GO, but the precise mechanisms responsible for the orbital damage remains to be elucidated. The autoimmune and inflammatory nature of GO has led to consider therapeutic approaches aimed at suppressing the immune response or at abating the inflammatory process. In this regard, immunosuppressive therapy is widely employed in patients with moderate to severe GO. Glucocorticoids, orbital radiotherapy, or a combination of both, are the most frequently used immunosuppressive therapies, but other treatments like cyclosporine, azathioprine, intravenous immunoglobulins, and plasma exchange, have also been used (Table 1).

1.   GLUCOCORTICOIDS

Glucocorticoids have gained an established place in the management of GO in view of their anti-inflammatory and immunosuppressive actions.[2] These include: i) interference with T and B lymphocyte functions, ii) reduction in the recruitment of neutrophils, monocytes and macrophage into the inflamed area, iii) inhibition of the function of immunocompetent cells, iv) inhibition of the release of cytokines.[3] In addition glucocortoids decrease the synthesis and release of glycosaminoglycans by orbital fibroblasts.[4] Glucocorticoids have been used in GO patients since the early 1950s and have been administered either by local (retrobulbar or subconjunctival), or systemic (oral or intravenous) routes.[5] More recently the systemic use of glucocorticoids has also been proposed to prevent a progression that may occur in a minority of patients with mild ophthalmopathy after treatment with radioiodine for Graves' hyperthyroidism.[6]

Table 1. Immunosuppressive therapy in Graves' ophthalmopathy

Glucocorticoids
- Systemic
Oral
Intravenous
- Local
Retrobulbar or subconjunctival
Orbital radiotherapy
Immunosuppressive drugs
Cyclosporin A
Azathioprine
Cyclophosphamide
Pentoxyfilline
Intravenous immunoglobulins
Plasmapheresis
Somatostatin analogs
Cytokine antagonists

1.1   Oral glucocorticoids

Oral glucocorticoids (prednisone, prednisolone, methylprednisolone) are usually used at high doses to achieve a substantial immunosuppressive effect (initial dose: 60-100 mg/day prednisone or equivalent doses of other steroids, with subsequent tapering).[7] The treatment should last for several months (4-6) to abate the inflammatory process and to reduce the likelihood that eye manifestations may flare up upon reduction or drug withdrawal (Table 2). Oral glucocorticoids have proven to be particularly effective on optic neuropathy, soft tissue changes, and eye muscle motility disturbances: overall favorable responses are seen in about 60% of cases (Table 3).[8-15] The effects of treatment become evident after a few weeks or even days. Proptosis and longstanding extraocular muscle involvement respond poorly and require rehabilitative surgery.

The association with either orbital radiotherapy,[9] or cyclosporine,[10,13] would appear to be advantageous compared to the use of oral glucocorticoids alone (Fig. 1). In a randomized prospective study in patients with moderate to severe ophthalmopathy Bartalena *et al.*[9] showed excellent or good responses in 10/12 patients treated by combined therapy (radiotherapy and oral glucocorticoids) and in only 4/12 given glucocorticoids alone. Similarly, Kahaly et al.[10] reported a significant improvement in all signs of GO in 20 patients treated with oral prednisone (50-100 mg/day) for 10 weeks. Recurrences occurred in 8 patients, whereas, no recurrences were observed in another group of 20 patients who received cyclosporine concomitantly with glucocorticoids.[10] In a randomized study by Prummel et al.,[13] 11/18 (61%) patients responded to prednisone treatment, while only 4/12 (22%) improved after cyclosporine. Interestingly, the addition of cyclosporine to prednisone resulted in a favorable response in 5 of the 9 (56%) non-responders to prednisone alone; *vice versa*, the addition of prednisone to cyclosporine was associated with an improvement of the ophthalmopathy in 8 of the 14 (62%) nonresponders to cyclosporine alone. [13]

Table 2. Therapeutic immunosuppressive regimens for Graves' ophthalmopathy.

Therapy	Initial dose	Duration of therapy
Glucocorticoids		
Oral prednisone (1)	60-100 mg / day	4-6 months
I.V. methylprednisolone	0.5-1.0 g for 3 days	3-7 x at weekly intervals
Local methylprednisolone acetate(1)	10-40 mg	10-14 x at 20-30 day intervals
Cyclosporine (2)	5-10 mg / kg / d	2-6 months
Plasmapheresis (3)		4-12 sessions
Octreotide analogs	0.2-1.0 mg / d	3 months
I.V. Immunoglobulins	400-1000 mg / kg	2-5 times every 3 weeks for 4-5 months

(1) alone or with radiotherapy; (2) more effective when combined with glucocorticoids; (3) often combined with azathioprine, cyclophosphamide and glucocorticoids.

The efficacy of oral glucocorticoids is similar to that of orbital radiotherapy. In a prospective double-blind randomized clinical trial in patients with moderate ophthalmopathy favorable responses were observed in 47% of patients treated with radiotherapy (20 Gy) and in 50% of those treated with prednisone (60 mg daily for 2 weeks with gradual tapering of the dose to zero in eighteen weeks).[14] The response to prednisone was faster than that to radiotherapy, but both modalities were associated with similar responses in the different eye manifestations. The major drawback of oral glucocorticoids are the possible side effects. Most patients develop transient Cushingoid features, but the prevalence of other adverse effects, such as diabetes, depression, infections, peptic ulcer, hirsutism, hypertension is lower. This underscores the need for a careful selection of patients to be treated by oral glucocorticoids and for their careful follow-up.

Table 3. Results of commonly used immunosuppressive treatments for Graves' ophthalmopathy. (1) Combined with corticosteroids.

Therapy	Author	Year	Ref	Number of patients	Number of responders (%)
Oral glucocorticoids					
	Brown	1963	8	19	15 (80%)
	Bartalena	1983	9	12	5 (42%)
	Kahaly	1986	20	10	12 (60%)
	Wiersinga	1988	44	15	29 (64%)
	Prummel	1989	12	18	11 (61%)
	Prummel	1993	14	28	14 (50%)
	Kung	1996	12	10	6 (60%)
	Kahaly	1996	11	19	12 (63%)
				131	*104 (79%)*
Oral glucocorticoids + Radiotherapy					
	Bartalena	1983	9	36	26 (72%)
	Marcocci	1987	26	13	9 (64%)
				49	*35 (71%)*
I.V. glucocorticoids					
	Nagayama	1987	16	5	3 (60%)
	Kendall-Taylor	1988	17	11	8 (73%)
	Dandona	1989	18	37	32 (86%)
	Guy	1989	19	5	5 (100%)
	Hiromatsu	1994	20	15	12 (80%)
	Tagami	1996	21	27	27 (100%)
				100	*87 (87%)*
Somatostatin analogs					
	Chang	1992	55	6	6 (100%)
	Krassas	1995	56	12	7 (58%)
	Kung	1996	12	8	5 (62%)
	Krassas	1997	58	5	5 (100%)
				31	*23 (74%)*
Cyclosporine					
	Weetman	1983	36	2	2 (100%)
	Witte	1985	38	13	?
	Kahaly (1)	1986	10	20	19 (95%)
	Prummel	1989	13	18	4 (22%)
				40	*25 (63%)*

1.2   Intravenous glucocorticoids

In the last 10 years intravenous glucocorticoid pulse therapy (0.5-1 g) has been used in several studies (Tables 2 and 3). Various regimens have been used. The original protocol proposed by Nagayama *et al.*[16] consisted of the administration of 1 g methylprednisolone acetate for 3 consecutive days, which was repeated 3-7 times at weekly intervals (with a cumulative dose of 9-21g). This schedule, with modifications concerning the dose and the treatment interval, has been employed by various authors. In some cases oral glucocorticoids are given after the completion of the intravenous therapy.[16-21] It is worth noting that in one study five patients with optic neuropathy showed a substantial improvement in visual acuity within one week.[19]

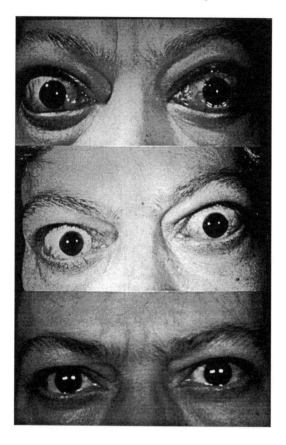

Figure 1. Eye changes before (upper panel), at 3 months (middle panel), and at 6 months (lower panel) treatment with orbital radiotherapy combined with high dose systemic glucocorticoids. (Reproduced with permission from the patient).

Pulses are remarkably well tolerated and possibly associated with fewer adverse effects, although hyperglycemia, hypertension, infections and gastric erosion have been described.[22] On the other hand the intravenous administration is more laborious than the oral route. The efficacy of pulse therapy appears to be slightly superior to that of oral glucocorticoids, but no randomized clinical trials comparing the two routes of glucocorticoid administration have been done so far.

1.3   Local glucocorticoids

The potential risks of systemic glucocorticoids prompted the evaluation of local (retrobulbar or subconjunctival) glucocorticoid therapy. This treatment consists of repeated injections of a methylprednisolone acetate over a period of several months (Table 2). Garber[23] reported an improvement of ocular conditions in 15 patients, being evident in most cases after the first injections. Subsequent studies have shown less favorable responses.[24,25] The effects of combined treatment with orbital radiotherapy and retrobulbar glucocorticoids (14 injections of 40 mg methylprednisolone acetate at 3-4 week interval) were prospectively evaluated in 44 patients: excellent or good results were observed in 11 patients (25%) compared to 60% of patients treated by orbital radiotherapy and systemic glucocorticoids.[26] Side effects of local therapy were limited to local discomfort and conjunctival hemorrhages in few instances. Thus, local glucocorticoid therapy appears to be less effective than systemic glucocorticoids, and therefore should be considered only in patients with contraindications to the use of systemic glucocorticoids.

2.   ORBITAL RADIOTHERAPY

Orbital radiotherapy has been used in the management of GO for almost 60 years.[27] The rationale for the use of orbital radiotherapy resides in its nonspecific anti-inflammatory effect and in the high radiosensitivity of retrobulbar lymphocytes, especially activated helper T cells.[28] Compiling the results of 11 studies, beneficial effects were reported in 228/351 (65%) cases, a percentage similar to that observed with oral prednisone.[29] Favorable effects of orbital irradiation have been reported especially on soft tissue inflammatory changes, extraocular muscle involvement, but also on optic neuropathy.[30] At variance, proptosis appeared to be less responsive to treatment. The therapeutic use of orbital radiotherapy is extensively discussed in Chapter 8.

3.   PLASMAPHERESIS

The use of plasmapheresis has been proposed on the premise that, as in other autoimmune disease, such as myasthenia gravis and Goodpasture's syndrome, removal of either autoantibodies or immune complexes might be beneficial for GO. This procedure has been used mostly in combination with immunosuppressive drugs (azathioprine, cyclophosphamide, and oral glucocorticoids) (Table 2). Favorable results have been reported by several investigators in non-controlled studies.[31-33] In a prospective controlled study the addition of plasmapheresis to prednisone and azathioprine was found to be more effective than the use of the immunosuppressive regimen alone.[34] In another study, plasma exchange without glucocorticoids administration was found to be ineffective.[35] Thus it would appear that plasmapheresis is effective only if combined with other immunosuppressive drugs. Its use should be considered when all other therapeutic regimens have failed.

4.   IMMUNOSUPPRESSIVE DRUGS

Cyclosporine has been the most widely used immunosuppressive drug in the management of GO (Table 2). The first report on its use in GO showed a favorable response,[36] but subsequent open trials gave conflicting results.[37, 38] In a randomized clinical trial comparing the efficacy of a 12-week course of prednisone with cyclosporine, Prummel *et al.*[13] reported a higher success rate in the prednisone group (61%) than in the cyclosporine group (22%). In patients with unsatisfactory results the combination of 20 mg prednisone with cyclosporine for an additional 12-week period resulted in a success rate of 59%. Cyclosporine was better tolerated than prednisone. In another randomized study the association of cyclosporine with oral prednisone was more effective that prednisone alone.[10] Both studies showed a greater efficacy of cyclosporine when combined with prednisone than either treatment used alone. The efficacy of the combination therapy has a sound theoretical foundation, since prednisone can destroy clones of effector lymphocytes, whereas cyclosporine prevents their reemergence.[2] Thus it can be concluded that monotherapy with cyclosporine is not indicated. Its use, combined with prednisone, can be considered in patients with no response to prednisone alone.

Several other immunosuppressive drugs have been employed in the management of GO. *Azathioprine* produced little beneficial effects in an open trial,[39] and in a more recent controlled study.[40] In a uncontrolled study *cyclophosphamide* has been reported to produce some improvement of soft tissue changes.[41] *Ciamexone* initially showed some favorable effects,[42] which were not confirmed in a controlled study.[43] Recently *pentoxyfilline*, an *in vitro* inhibitor of glycosaminoglycan production by orbital fibroblasts, has been used in 10 patients with beneficial effects on soft tissue changes in 8 of them.[44]

The latest therapeutic suggestion among immunomodulatory treatments might be the use of *cytokine antagonists*.[45] Cytokines exert several actions that may be relevant to the pathogenesis of Graves' ophthalmopathy.[46] *In vitro* studies have shown that cytokines induce the expression of HLA class

II molecules and heath shock proteins. Moreover they stimulate the proliferation of human retroorbital fibroblasts and the synthesis and secretion of glycosaminoglycans.[46] Tan *et al.*[47] have recently shown that interleukin (IL)-1 receptor antagonists and soluble IL-1 receptor inhibit the glycosaminoglycan synthesis and secretion by cultured human orbital fibroblasts from patients with Graves' ophthalmopathy. This study provides the rational for a novel approach to the treatment of Graves' ophthalmopathy by using cytokine antagonists that might interfere with the ongoing inflammatory reactions in the retroorbital space. In this regard it is worth noting that higher serum levels of IL-1 receptor antagonists were found to correlate with a favorable response to orbital radiotherapy.[48] No data are presently available on the use of IL-1 or other cytokine antagonists in Graves' ophthalmopathy.

5.   INTRAVENOUS IMMUNOGLOBULINS

High-dose intravenous immunoglobulins (IVIG) has been favorably used in several autoimmune diseases. Their beneficial effect can be mediated by several mechanisms, including blocking of idiotypic epitopes by anti-idiotypic antibodies, inhibition of cytokine release, down-regulation of immune-competent cells. It has recently been suggested that the beneficial effect of IVIG in autoimmune diseases may be due to the finding that almost all IVIG preparations contain TGF-ß, an effective immunosuppressive cytokine.[49]

Antonelli *et al.*[50] treated 14 patients with IVIG alone or in combination with orbital radiotherapy and compared the results with a "historical" group treated with oral glucocorticoid and orbital irradiation. Improvement was observed in all three groups, without significant differences among them. In a subsequent randomized study IVIG resulted in a positive response in 62% of patients compared to a response rate of 63% in patients treated by glucocorticoids.[11] These data were confirmed in another prospective, not randomized study.[51] The beneficial effects occurred on soft tissue inflammatory changes, proptosis, and extraocular muscle involvement. At variance with these favorable results, Seppel *et al.*[52] reported no significant changes in ocular involvement in 10 patients treated with IVIG. In summary, the results of IVIG therapy on GO are similar to those obtained with standard treatments, such as orbital radiotherapy and glucocorticoids. Although the reported side effects were rather limited, the potential risk for transmitting infectious agents and the high cost of this treatment must be taken into account.

6.   SOMATOSTATIN ANALOGS

Orbital uptake of $[^{111}$In-DTPA-D-Phe$^1]$-octreotide can be observed *in vivo* in the orbital tissue of patients with GO,[53] with a higher orbital uptake in patients with active ophthalmopathy compared to those with inactive eye disease.[54] Moreover, specific treatment of GO may decrease the uptake.[54] Thus, it was postulated that positive a octreoscan might reflect the activity of the ophthalmopathy and predict its response to treatment.

The somatostatin analogue, octreotide, was first used in GO patients by Chang *et al.*,[55] who showed an improvement of extraocular muscle function and soft tissue involvement in 6 patients (Table 2). In a prospective study, Krassas *et al.*,[56] using the same treatment schedule, reported positive results in 7 of 12 patients, with no effects in the remaining 5 patients. Interestingly, octreoscans were positive in those patients who had a favorable therapeutic response, but negative in all but one in whom octreotide treatment was a failure.[56] Kung *et al.*[12] compared the effects of octreotide (0.6 mg/day for 3 months) with those achieved with glucocorticoids. Although octreotide decreased soft tissue inflammation and improved eye symptoms, glucocorticoid treatment resulted in a greater reduction in the activity score and a more marked effect on extraocular muscle.[12] Durak *et al.*[57] used higher doses of octreotide (1 mg/day for 3 months), but were unable to observe any favorable effect of the drug on the ophthalmopathy. Favorable responses were recently reported in 5 GO patients using lanreotide, a new long-acting somatostatin analogue.[58]

In the above studies, side effects of somatostatin analogue therapy were in general limited to mild gastrointestinal symptoms occurring during the first week of treatment.

The mechanism of action of somatostatin analogues is not fully understood. Somatostatin may inhibit several important functions, such as the local release of IGF-I[59] or cytokines,[60] that appear to be relevant in triggering and/or maintaining the ongoing reactions in the retroorbital tissues of patients with ophthalmopathy.

Only few studies have been performed so far, and the number of treated patients is limited. Therefore, it is difficult to draw definite and sound conclusions on the real effectiveness of somatostatin analogues. Properly controlled studies enrolling a larger number of patients are warranted.

7.   OTHER TREATMENTS

Bromocriptine has occasionally been reported to have beneficial effects in forms of GO resistant to conventional treatments.[61] This effect has been attributed to a possible antiproliferative effect on immunocompetent T lymphocytes. A transient benefit has been reported in a few patients treated with metrodinazole.[62] The beneficial effects of acupuncture, suggested by a Chinese study,[63] were not confirmed in a more recent randomized study.[64]

8.   CONCLUSIONS

Several immunosuppressive approaches are currently available to treat Graves' ophthalmopathy. Reviewing the existing alternatives it appears that no treatment is more effective than systemic glucocorticoid or orbital radiotherapy, and possibly their combination. The use of intravenous glucocorticoids is promising and seems worthwhile in emergency situations, but it remains to be established whether this route of administration bears clear advantages over the oral administration in terms of effectiveness and side effects.

A substantial proportion of patients (20-40%) respond only partially or not at all to immunosuppressive treatment. It is conceivable that the effectiveness of treatment may be improved by properly selecting patients who are prone to have beneficial results, i.e. those with a high degree of disease activity, with ophthalmopathy of recent onset and/or recent progression. Only in a limited number of cases the results of treatment are really satisfactory but the majority will still need rehabilitative surgery. In these cases treatment should aim at inactivation of the disease in order to allow orbital surgery as soon as possible.

9.   REFERENCES

1. Burch HB, Wartofsky L. Graves' ophthalmopathy: current concepts regarding pathogenesis and management. Endocr Rev 1993; 14:747-793.
2. Wiersinga WM. 1990 Immunosuppressive treatment of Graves' ophthalmopathy. Trends Endocrinol Metab 1990; 1:377.
3. Bartalena L, Marcocci C, Bogazzi F, Bruno-Bossio G, Pinchera A. Glucocorticoid therapy of Graves' ophthalmopathy. Exp Clin Endocrinol 1991; 97:320-327.
4. Smith TJ, Bahn RS, Gorman CA. 1989 Hormonal regulation of hyaluronate synthesis in cultured fibroblasts; evidence for differences between retroocular and dermal fibroblasts. J Clin Endocrinol Metab 1989; 69:1019
5. Bartalena L, Marcocci C, Pinchera A. 1997 Treating severe Graves' ophthalmopathy. Bailliere's Clin Endocrinol Metab 1997; 11:521.
6. Bartalena L, Marcocci C, Bogazzi F, et al. Relation between therapy for hyperthyroidism and the course of Graves' ophthalmopathy. N Engl J Med 1998; 338:73.
7. McConaey WM. Medical therapy. In: Gorman CA Waller RR Dyer JA, eds. The Eye and Orbit in Thyroid Disease. New York: Raven Press 1984: 317.

8. Brown K, Coburn JW, Wigod RA, Hiss JM, Dowling JT. Adrenal steroid therapy of severe infiltrative ophthalmopathy of Graves' disease. Am J Med 1963; 34:786.
9. Bartalena L, Marcocci C, Chiovato L, *et al*. Orbital cobalt irradiation combined with systemic corticosteroids for Graves' ophthalmopathy: comparison with systemic corticosteroids alone. J Clin Endocrinol Metab 1983; 56:1139.
10. Kahaly G, Schrezenmeir J, Krause U, Schweikert B, Meuer S, Muller W. Ciclosporin and prednisone v. prednisone in treatment of Graves' ophthalmopathy: a controlled, randomized and prospective study. Eur J Clin Invest 1986; 16:415.
11. Kahaly G, Pitz S, Muller-Forell W, Hommel G. Randomized trial of intravenous immunoglobulins *versus* prednisolone in Graves' ophthalmopathy. Clin Exp Immunol 1996; 106:197.
12. Kung AWC, Michon J, Tai KS, Chan FL. The effect of somatostatin versus corticosteroid in the treatment of Graves' ophthalmopathy. Thyroid 1996; 6:381.
13. Prummel MF, Mourits MP, Berghout A, *et al*. Prednisone and cyclosporine in the treatment of severe Graves' ophthalmopathy. N Engl J Med 1989; 321:1353.
14. Prummel MF, Mourits MP, Blank L, Berghout A, Koornneef L, Wiersinga WM. Randomised double-blind trial of prednisone versus radiotherapy in Graves' ophthalmopathy. Lancet 1993; 342:949.
15. Wiersinga WM, Smit T, Schuster-Uittenhoeve ALJ, van der Gaag R, Koornneef L. Therapeutic outcome of prednisone medication and orbital irradiation in patients with Graves' ophthalmopathy. Ophthalmologica 1988; 197:75.
16. Nagayama Y, Izumi M, Kiriyama T, *et al*. Treatment of Graves' ophthalmopathy with high-dose intravenous methylprednisolone pulse therapy. Acta Endocrinol (Copenh) 1987; 116:513.
17. Kendall-Taylor P, Crombie AL, Stephenson AM, Hardwick M, Hall K. Intravenous methylprednisolone in the treatment of Graves' ophthalmopathy. Br Med J 1988; 297:1574.
18. Dandona P, Havard CWH, Mier A. Methylprednisolone and Graves' ophthalmopathy. Br Med J 1989; 298:830.
19. Guy JR, Fagien S, Donovan JP, Rubin ML. Methylprednisolone pulse therapy in severe dysthyroid optic neuropathy. Ophthalmology 1989; 96:1048.
20. Hiromatsu Y, Tanaka K, Sato M, *et al*. Intravenous methylprednisolone pulse therapy for Graves' ophthalmopathy. Endocrine J 1993; 40:63.
21. Tagami T, Tanaka K, Sugawa H, *et al*. High-dose intravenous steroid pulse therapy in thyroid-associated ophthalmopathy. Endocrine J 1996; 43:689.
22. Baethge BA, Lidsky MD, Goldberg JW. A study of the adverse effects of high-dose intravenous (pulse) methylprednisolone therapy in patients with rheumatic disease. Ann Pharmacotherapy 1992; 96:316.
23. Garber MI. Methylprednisolone in the treatment of exophthalmos. Lancet 1966; 1:958.
24. Riley. Discussion of the paper by Ivy HK, Medical approach to ophthalmopathy of Graves' disease. Mayo Clin Proc 1972; 47:992.
25. Trobe JD, Glaser JS, Laflamme P. Dysthyroid optic neuropathy. Arch Ophthalmol 1978; 96:1199.
26. Marcocci C, Bartalena L, Panicucci M, *et al*. Orbital cobalt irradiation combined with retrobulbar or systemic corticosteroids for Graves' ophthalmopathy: a comparative study. Clin Endocrinol 1987; 27:33.
27. Pinchera A, Bartalena L, Chiovato L, Marcocci C. Radiotherapy of Graves' ophthalmopathy. In: Gorman CA, Waller RR, Dyer JA, eds. The Eye and Orbit in Thyroid Disease. New York: Raven Press 1984; 301.

28. Marcocci C, Bartalena L, Bruno-Bossio G, *et al*. Orbital radiotherapy in the treatment of endocrine ophthalmopathy: when and why? In: Kahaly G, ed. Endocrine Ophthalmopathy - Molecular, Immunological and Clinical Aspects. Basel: Karger 1993: 131.

29. Wiersinga WM. Advances in medical therapy of thyroid associated ophthalmopathy. Orbit 1996; 15:177.

30. Bartalena L, Marcocci C, Manetti L, *et al*. Orbital radiotherapy for Graves' ophthalmopathy. Thyroid 1998; 8:439.

31. Dandona P, Marshall NJ, Bidey SP, Nathan A, Havard CWH. Exophthalmos and pretibial myxoedema not responding to plasmapheresis. Br Med J 1979; 2:667.

32. Glinoer D, Etienne-Decerf J, Schrooven M, *et al*. 1986 Beneficial effects of intensive plasma exchange followed by immunosuppressive therapy in severe Graves' ophthalmopathy. Acta Endocrinol (Copenh) 1986; 111:30.

33. Berlin G, Hjelm H, Lieden G, Tegler L. Plasma exchange in endocrine ophthalmopathy. J Clin Apheresis 1990; 5:192.

34. De Rosa G, Menichella G, Della S, *et al*. Plasma exchange in Graves' ophthalmopathy. Prog Clin Biol Res 1990; 337:321.

35. Kelly W, Longson D, Smithard D, *et al*. An evaluation of plasma exchange for Graves' ophthalmopathy. Clin Endocrinol 1983; 18:485.

36. Weetman AP, McGregor AM, Ludgate M, *et al*. Cyclosporin improves Graves' ophthalmopathy. Lancet 1983; 2:486.

37. Brabant G, Peter H, Becker H, Schwarzrock R, Wonigeit K, Hesch RD. 1984 Cyclosporin in infiltrative eye disease. Lancet. 1984; 1:515.

38. Witte A, Landgraf R, Markl A, Boergen K-P, Hasenfratz G, Pickardt CR. Treatment of Graves' ophthalmopathy with cyclosporin A. Klin Wochenschr 1985; 63:1000.

39. Burrow GN, Mitchell MS, Howard RMO, Morrow LB. Immunosuppressive therapy for the eye changes of Graves' disease. J Clin Endocriol Metab 1970; 31:307.

40. Perros P, Weightman DR, Crombie AL, Kendall-Taylor P. Azathioprine in the treatment of thyroid-associated ophthalmopathy. Acta Endocrinol (Copenh) 1990; 122:8.

41. Bigos ST, Nisula BC, Daniels GH, Eastman RC, Johnston HH, Kohler PO. Cyclophosphamide in the management of advanced Graves' ophthalmopathy. A preliminary report. Ann Intern Med 1979; 90:921.

42. Utech C, Wulle KG, Panitz N, Kiefer H. Treatment of Graves' ophthalmopathy with new immunosuppressive agents. Dev Ophthalmol 1989; 20:109.

43. Kahaly G, Lieb W, Muller-Forell W, *et al*. Ciamexone in endocrine orbitopathy: a randomized, double-blind, placebo-controlled study. Acta Endocrinol (Copenh) 1990; 122:13.

44. Balazs C, Kiss E, Vamos A, Molnar I, Farid NR. Beneficial effect of pentoxifilline on thyroid associated ophthalmopathy (TAO): A pilot study. J Clin Endocrinol Metab 1998; 82:1999.

45. Bartalena L, Marcocci C, Pinchera A. Editorial: Cytokine antagonist: New ideas for the management of Graves' ophthalmopathy. J Clin Endocrinol Metab 1996; 81:446.

46. Heufelder AE. Pathogenesis of Graves' ophthalmopathy: recent controversies and progress. Eur J Endocrinol 1995; 132:532.

47. Tan GH, Dutto CM, Bahn RS. Interleukin-1 receptor antagonist and soluble interleukin-1 receptor inhibit interleukin-1-induced glycosaminoglycan production in cultured human orbital fibroblasts from patients with Graves' ophthalmopathy. J Clin Endocrinol Metab 1996; 81:449.

48. Hofbauer LC, Muhlberg T, Konig A, Heufelder G, Schworm H-D, Heufelder AE. Soluble interleukin-1 receptor antagonist serum levels in smokers and nonsmokers with Graves' ophthalmopathy undergoing orbital radiotherapy. J Clin Endocrinol Metab 1997; 82:2244.

49. Kekow J, Reinhold D, Pap T, Ansorge S. Intravenous immunoglobulins and transforming growth factor B. Lancet 1998; 351:184.

50. Antonelli A, Saracino A, Alberti B, *et al*. High-dose intravenous immunoglobulin treatment in Graves' ophthalmopathy. Acta Endocrinol (Copenh) 1992; 126:13.

51. Baschieri L, Antonelli A, Nardi S, *et al*. Intravenous immunoglobulin versus corticosteroid in treatment of Graves' ophthalmopathy. Thyroid 1997; 7:579.

52. Seppel T, Schlaghecke R, Becker A, Engelbrecht V, Feldkamp J, Kornely E. High-dose intravenous therapy with 7S immunoglobulins in autoimmune endocrine ophthalmopathy. Clin Exp Rheumatol 1996; 14 (Suppl 15): S109.

53. Krenning EP, Kwekkeboom DJ, Bakker WH, *et al*. Somatostatin receptor scintigraphy with [^{111}In-DTPA-D-Phe^1]- and [^{123}I-Tyr^3]-octreotide: the Rotterdam experience with more than 1000 patients. Eur J Nucl Med 1993 20:716.

54. Kahaly G, Diaz M, Hahn K, Beyer J, Bockisch A. Indium-111-pentreotide scintigraphy in Graves' ophthalmopathy. J Nucl Med 1995; 36:550.

55. Chang TC, Kao SCS, Huang KM. Octreotide and Graves' ophthalmopathy and pretibial myxoedema. Br Med J 1992; 304:158.

56. Krassas GE, Dumas A, Pontikides N, Kaltsas T. Somatostatin receptor scintigraphy and octreotide treatment in patients with thyroid eye disease. Clin Endocrinol 1995; 42:571.

57. Durak I, Durak H, Ergin M, Yurekli Y, Kaynak S. Somatostatin receptors in the orbit. Clin Nucl Med 1995; 20:237.

58. Krassas GE, Kaltsas T, Dumas A, Pontikides N, Tolis G. Lanreotide in the treatment of patients with thyroid eye disease. Eur J Endocrinol 1997; 136:416.

59. Hansson HA, Petruson B, Skottnerm A. Somatomedin C in the pathogenesis of malignant exophthalmos of endocrine origin. Lancet 1986; 1:218.

60. Bahn RS, Heufelder AE. Pathogenesis of Graves' ophthalmopathy. N Engl J Med. 1993; 329:1468.

61. Kolodziej-Maciejewska H, Reterski Z. Positive effect of bromocriptine treatment in Graves' disease orbitopathy. Exp Clin Endocrinol 1985; 86:241.

62. Harden R, Chisolm C, Cant J. The effect of metrodinazole on thyroid function and exophthalmos in man. Ophthalmology 1967; 16.

63. Zesen W, Shubai J, Zutong Z. The effect of acupuncture in 40 cases of endocrine ophthalmopathy. J Trad Chinese Med 1985; 5:19.

64. Rogvi-Hansen B, Perrild H, Christensen T, Detmar S, Siersbaek-Nielsen K, Hansen J. Acupuncture in the treatment of Graves' ophthalmopathy. A blinded randomized study. Acta Endocrinol (Copenh) 191; 124:143.

Chapter 8

Radiotherapy for Graves' ophthalmopathy

George J. Kahaly,* Colum A. Gorman, Henk B. Kal, Maarten Ph. Mourits,
Aldo Pinchera, H. Stevie Tan, Mark F. Prummel.
*Department of Endocrinology/Metabolism, Building 303, Johannes Gutenberg Klinikum,
University of Mainz, 55101-Mainz, Germany

1. INTRODUCTION

The interest in the treatment of benign diseases with radiation therapy has grown particularly in the Western part of the world. In 1996, a questionnaire was sent to 1348 institutes worldwide listed in the directory of the Society for Therapeutic Radiology and Oncology asking whether the respondents considered a list of 28 most common benign disorders as being a good indication for orbital radiotherapy.[1] Questions concerned the frequency of such treatments and the treatment schedules used. The prevention of keloid formation was the most widely accepted indication, followed by Graves' ophthalmopathy. Thus, radiotherapy for this orbital disorder is generally accepted and applied worldwide.

Radiation therapy for Graves' ophthalmopathy has been used since 1913.[2] The prevailing theory in the 1940s was that the pituitary produced hormonal factors that caused exophthalmos,[3] and radiotherapy was thus aimed at this gland. The older radiation delivery systems were poorly collimated and easily led to inadvertent orbital irradiation.[4] It appeared, that only those patients with inadvertent orbital irradiation showed improvement.[5] In the mean time, recognizing the sensitivity of orbital lymphocytes to radiation, the direction of therapy moved to selective irradiation of the retrobulbar structures, excluding the pituitary gland from the treatment field. The advent of well-collimated irradiation allowed the treatment to be optimally delivered to the orbit.

The rationale for the use of orbital radiotherapy resides in the well established radiosensitivity of lymphocytes that infiltrate the orbit and are considered important effectors in this disorder.[6,7] The histologic features of Graves' ophthalmopathy are characterized by marked edema and lymphocytic infiltration.[8-10] Recent studies indicate that activated orbital T-lymphocytes secrete cytokines, which in a paracrine manner are thought to induce glycosaminoglycan production by fibroblasts.[6] Excessive secretion of the hydrophilic molecules results in tissue edema, which, besides lymphocyte infiltration, causes the marked swelling of the tissues.[11,12]

2.   TECHNIQUE

Orbital radiotherapy can be delivered as waves either x-rays or gamma. The current measure of the radiation dose is the Gray (Gy); one Gy equals 100 rads. Most early radiotherapy, no longer used in ophthalmopathy, was delivered by low or orthovoltage (85-400 kV) machines.[13-16] These low-energy, poorly focussed modalities deposited most of the radiation at the skin surface and had preferential bone absorption. The orthovoltage equipment has now been replaced by telecobalt or megavoltage linear accelerators that allow delivery of a high-energy, low-scattered, and well-collimated beam to the retrobulbar space, avoiding undue irradiation of adjacent structures such as the lens, cornea, pituitary, and hypothalamus (Table 1). Today's preferred megavoltage (4 or 6 MeV) machines produce a photon beam that is sharply defined and using one field, skin sparing with a maximum dose of at least 0.5 cm from the skin surface.

Table 1. Actual technical modalities for orbital radiotherapy in patients with Graves' ophthalmopathy

	Linear accelerator	Telecobalt 60
Irradiation waves	4-6 MeV photons	Gamma rays
Irradiation field	6 x 5 cm	7 x 6 cm
Angle (degrees)	2	3
Source distance	100 cm	80 cm

Regardless of the delivery method, radiotherapy is given in fractionated daily doses to decrease damage to normal structures. In most institutions it is administered in standard total doses of 16 (Germany) to 20 Gy with a 6 MeV photo beam, divided into 8 to 10 daily fractions of 2 Gy over 2 weeks. Localization and verification films with lead markers on the eyelids of each eye are performed for each patient on a simulator. The posterior field border is located anterior to the sella turcica. The floor and the roof of the orbit represent the upper and lower border of the radiation field (Fig.1). The dose is calculated at the midline and given by two 2-3° posteriorly angled lateral portals of 6 x 5 cm (to avoid irradiation of the contralateral lens), with the patient's head fixed by a full head shell. Dose calculation is based on transversal CT scan slices of the orbit. The light point of the central beam is first positioned tangentially on both corneas and the table is then lifted for half of the field size plus the desired distance from the cornea. This is done in electronically controlled increments of 1 mm. Thus the anterior field margin lies 15 mm posterior to the plane of the cornea, which is a safe distance from the lens. Using telecobalt devices, which may produce more scatter and penumbra, the radiation field size can be doubled in a ventro-dorsal direction and brought to the final treatment volume by positioning a lead shield in the central beam axis, which then represents the anterior margin of the truly irradiated field.

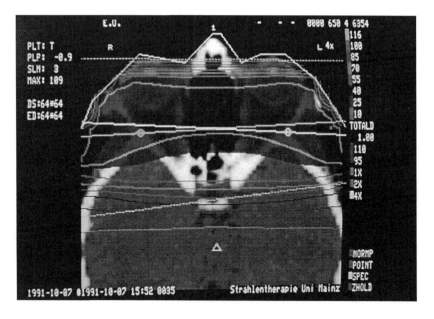

Figure 1. Irradiation field or target volume for orbital radiotherapy (Contributed by G.J. Kahaly).

3. CLINICAL TRIALS

There have been numerous uncontrolled studies of radiotherapy as second-line treatment in Graves' ophthalmopathy, with a reported response rate of approximately 60%.[17-20] However, many studies were retrospective, and in most the natural course towards improvement of eye changes could have influenced the results because of a long interval between treatment and assessment of outcome. Some patients were simultaneously treated with glucocorticoids,[21] or included despite an abnormal thyroid function, which can affect the severity of the eye changes.[22] A precise analysis of the results is difficult because of the often limited number of patients in individual studies, differences in radiotherapy procedures and doses, and the lack of definite criteria for the evaluation of ocular changes before and after therapy. Despite these limitations, it appears that favorable responses can be achieved in nearly two-thirds of the patients. Inflammatory soft tissue changes and extraocular muscle involvement of short duration are, in general, favorably affected, whereas proptosis and longstanding eye muscle involvement are relatively resistant to radiotherapy.[13,14,23]

3.1   Randomized studies

Orbital radiotherapy has been used in association with systemic high-dose corticosteroids to exploit the more rapid action of glucocorticoids and the more persistent effect of radiotherapy. In two randomized studies, Bartalena *et al.*, showed that the combined therapy was more effective than glucocorticoids alone, or than orbital radiotherapy alone, suggesting a possibly synergistic effect.[14,15] On the other hand, Prummel *et al.*,[24] reported that orbital radiotherapy and high-dose prednisone were equally effective in patients with moderately severe eye disease, with prednisone being slightly more effective on soft tissue changes and radiotherapy on eye muscle motility. In this double blind trial of prednisone *vs.* radiotherapy in patients with untreated moderately severe ophthalmopathy in whom euthyroidism was maintained throughout the study, patients were randomized to a 3-month course of oral prednisone and sham irradiation or to retrobulbar radiotherapy (20 Gy) and placebo capsules. A successful outcome, as assessed 24 weeks after the start of treatment according to predefined criteria, was observed in 50% of the prednisone treated and 46% of the irradiated patients. Therapeutic outcome was primarily determined by the change in the highest NO SPECS class. Successful treatment was largely caused by improvement in eye muscle motility and soft tissue swelling, and associated with a decrease in eye muscle enlargement on CT scan. There were no clinically important changes in proptosis. The degree of improvement was not different between the two treatment groups, but prednisone patients improved more rapidly. In the view of Prummel *et al.*, orbital radiotherapy and prednisone are equally effective as initial treatment in moderately severe Graves' ophthalmopathy.

Mourits *et al.*[25] presented a double blind randomized trial comparing retrobulbar radiotherapy (20 Gy over 2 weeks) *vs.* sham irradiation, and hypothesized that radiotherapy would not influence the course of the eye disease. Enrolled were euthyroid patients with class 4 grade a-c or, class 3 grade a-c, or class 2 grade b or c (in the worst eye), between 20-75 yr., without previous treatment, and with informed consent. Exclusion criteria were diabetes mellitus and dysthyroid optic neuropathy. Before treatment, at 4, 12 and 24 weeks after starting therapy, the NO SPECS classes, eyelid aperture and swelling, proptosis and eye muscle motility as well as total and subjective eye scores and clinical activity score were evaluated. Definition of outcome was as follows: a decrease in NO SPECS class or grade was regarded a success, an increase in class or grade a failure, whereas no decrease or increase were regarded as no change. According to this, a success was observed in 63% after radiotherapy *vs.* 31% for sham irradiation, no change in 30 *vs.* 52% and a failure was noted in 7 *vs.* 17%. Significant improvements for elevation of the globe, total and subjective eye scores, as well as clinical activity scores were seen after radiotherapy (Fig. 2). Whereas, significant deterioration of subjective eye and activity scores was seen in the sham group. In patients with NO SPECS class 4, 82% (radiotherapy) *vs.* 27% (sham) responded, but in class 2 or 3, no clear differences were noted (39 *vs.* 36%). Mourits *et al.* concluded that orbital radiotherapy improved eye motility and that this treatment is effective in patients with motility impairment, only.

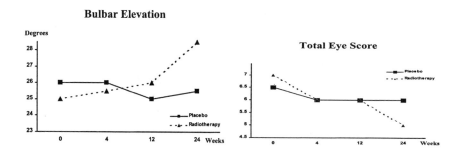

Figure 2. Elevation of the globe and Total Eye Score in patients with Graves' ophthalmopathy treated with radiotherapy or placebo.(Contributed by M.Ph. Mourits[25])

Gorman *et al.*[26] presented the results at 6 months of a double blind trial, where a *single* randomly selected orbit was treated with 20 Gy of supervoltage radiotherapy. Inclusion criteria were mild to moderate eye disease, euthyroidism either on therapy or without, over the age of 30 yr., willingness to omit all but local treatment measures for one year, and informed consent. Patients had to exhibit 3 of the following criteria: swollen eyelids or red swollen conjunctiva of the eye, staring or bulging eyes, double vision, involvement of both eyes, pain or excessive watering, and visible muscle enlargement on CT scan. Exclusion criteria were previous radiotherapy or surgical decompression, pregnancy, diabetes mellitus, steroid therapy within 2 weeks of starting, and optic neuropathy. Five fundamental measures before and after treatment were done: 1) volume of extraocular muscle, 2) volume of fat/connective tissue, 3) range of extraocular muscle motion in degrees on a perimeter 4) diplopia fields and 5) lid fissure width. In the treated and untreated orbit, changes from baseline in measures of orbital muscle and fat volume, proptosis, range of extraocular muscle motion, and area of diplopia fields at 3 and 6 months were compared. None of these parameters showed statistically significant differences between the treated and untreated orbit at either 3 or 6 months. Results at one year are pending. Since the baseline characteristics of the Mayo Clinic study are still not known definitive conclusions from the preliminary data cannot yet be drawn. It will be interesting to compare the final results between both randomized trials.

4.   LOW VERSUS HIGH DOSE RADIOTHERAPY

Radiation doses range from the typical high doses used for malignancies, to less than 1% of these doses in benign disorders. In most countries, a standard orbital radiotherapy dose of 20 Gy is delivered over two weeks (higher doses like 30 Gy do not provide further benefit), whereas in central Europe, especially in Germany, markedly lower radiotherapy doses, e.g. 4-10 Gy are administered.[16] Clinical and experimental data strongly suggest that low dose radiotherapy (single fractions of 1 Gy) is sufficient to achieve an antiphlogistic effect on acute and chronic inflammatory processes, like in insertion tendinitis and osteoarthritis, despite a complete lack of understanding of the biological mechanisms involved.[27] Therefore, it is very likely that different radiobiological mechanisms are involved at the higher and lower ends of the dose spectrum. There are no data provide evidence for the superiority of the higher dosages with respect to response and recurrence rates. Low dose orbital radiotherapy can be repeated in cases of recurrence, whereas with a second series of 20 Gy, the dose of tumor therapy is almost attained. Since it is important to reduce the radiation burden, it is attractive to reduce the total dose, especially if similar effectiveness could be proved.

Although orbital radiotherapy is a commonly used treatment for ophthalmopathy, controlled trials evaluating different dosages have not been done. A retrospective evaluation of high (20 Gy) and low dose (10 Gy) orbital radiotherapy in more than 100 patients was reported showing no significant differences in outcome.[28] Furthermore, a randomized trial was reported comparing three radiotherapy protocols in patients with moderately severe and clinically active eye disease.[28] Sixty two euthyroid patients with untreated eye disease, and no signs of optic neuropathy were enrolled. Orbital radiotherapy (telecobalt 60) was administered either in 20 fractions of 1 Gy weekly over 20 weeks (group A), or in 10 fractions of 1 Gy daily over 2 weeks (B), or in 10 fractions of 2 Gy/day/2 weeks (C). Before and 6 months after starting radiotherapy, ophthalmic investigation and MR imaging were performed. Therapeutic outcome was determined by changes in the highest NO SPECS class.

Therapeutic outcome

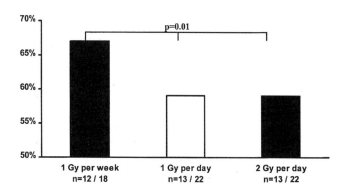

Figure 3. Successful therapeutic outcome in the three radiotherapy groups (Contributed by G.J. Kahaly[28])

A successful outcome was observed in 67% (A), 59% (B), and 59% (C) of the patients, respectively (fig. 3). Subjective and objective signs (fig. 4) regressed most in group A: median decrease of proptosis was -2 mm in A, -1.5 mm in B, and -1 mm in C. Visual acuity and eye muscle motility improved in group A only. Eye muscle volume decreased in all groups, significantly more in group A. Radiotherapy induced conjunctivitis was not observed in group A, but seen in 18% and 36% of B and C subjects (fig. 5).

Thus, in patients with moderately severe ophthalmopathy, the protracted 1Gy/week protocol was more effective and better tolerated than the shorter radiotherapy regimens, and subjective/objective ophthalmic signs decreased most in groups A (1 Gy/week) and B (1 Gy/day). This is in agreement with a study by Ravin *et al.*[29] who treated 37 patients with 10 fractionated doses of 1 Gy only. Muscle function in subjects with eye muscle abnormalities ameliorated but did not return to normal; visual function improved in all nine patients with optic neuropathy, although one still required decompression. There is experimental evidence that the clinically observed anti-inflammatory effects of low dose protracted radiotherapy, e.g. 1 Gy/week, are due to the functional alteration of cells involved in the inflammatory response.[27,30] A dose-dependent modulation of the nitric oxide pathway was observed with a significant inhibition by a low radiation dose, whereas a high dose resulted in a stimulation. Nitric oxide plays a central role in acute inflammation. It contributes to edema formation, increases the vascular permeability, and is involved in inflammatory pain.

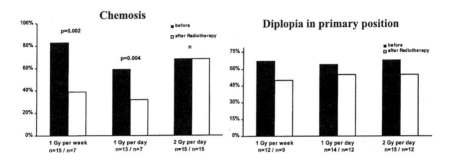

Figure 4. Graves' ophthalmopathy patients with chemosis, and diplopia in primary position before and at 6 months after the three different radiotherapy regimens (Contributed by G.J. Kahaly[28])

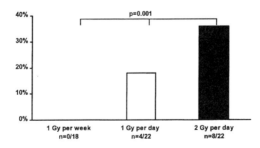

Figure 5. Radiation induced conjunctivitis in the three radiotherapy regimens (Contributed by G.J. Kahaly[28])

The effects of low-dose irradiation have also been studied in two rat models of inflammatory monoarticular arthritis. A fractionated dose schedule of four times 1 Gy over 4 days had a therapeutic effect, with a significant reduction in bone resorption and cartilage glycosaminoglycan loss in zymosan-induced arthritis and an anti-inflammatory effect in Mycobacterium tuberculosis-induced arthritis.[31] Thus, the suppressive interference of low and protracted doses of radiotherapy with the nitric oxide pathway may be one of the radiobiological mechanisms that underlies the clinically documented efficacy of anti-inflammatory radiotherapy. Radiation-induced reductions in nitric oxide production might result in the reduction of inflammatory edema as well as in pain relief.

5.   SMOKING AND RADIOTHERAPY

It was recently suggested that pretreatment serum levels of soluble interleukin-1 receptor antagonist (IL-1RA) may predict the therapeutic response to orbital radiotherapy, because low baseline IL-1RA values and an impaired surge after radiotherapy was associated with unfavorable responses to treatment.[32] This was especially evident in smokers. In a study from Pisa including 150 patients with clinically active ophthalmopathy,[33] a good response was seen more often in nonsmokers (61/65, 94%), than in smokers (58/85, 68%). Nevertheless, several smokers had excellent or good responses to irradiation. In accordance to this, at the endocrine outpatient clinic of the Mainz University Hospital, less than 60% of the ophthalmopathy patients are smokers. Although extensively informed, patients kept smoking during a randomized, prospective, single blind trial comparing different doses and application forms of orbital radiotherapy.[28] Still the response in smokers and nonsmokers was similar. This implies that cigarette smoking is only one of many risk factors involved in the progression of this thyroid-associated eye disease. Identification of such risk factors should be a goal of future research so that therapy may be improved and disease may be prevented.

6.   SAFETY

When radiation is well collimated, the risk of cataroctogenesis and oncogenesis appears to be low. Radiation tolerance dose for the lens is 10 Gy (covered), the optic nerve 50 Gy (safe), and for the retina 30-35 Gy (borderline safe).[34] Radiation doses necessary to induce cataract in subjects with ophthalmopathy are 2 and 5.5 Gy for single and fractionated radiotherapy, respectively.[16] The Stanford group did not detect any serious complications in their extended series after 21 years of follow-up.[35,36] Prevalence of retinopathy in the nondiabetic population approximates 8% according to the Beaver Dam eye study with 4311 subjects aged 43-84 yr. In this study, retinopathy was present in 10.7% hypertensive and 6.3% normotensive subjects, respectively.[34] Radiation retinopathy typically manifests between six months and three years after ophthalmic irradiation.[37] It is characterized by cotton-wool spots and intraretinal hemorrhages and exudates. Flurorescein angiography shows significant capillary nonperfusion in affected areas of the retina. Vascular changes in radiation retinopathy are divided in 5 classes: 1) focal endothelial cell loss in capillaries, 2) focal capillary occlusion with microaneurysms and hemorrhages, 3) capillary leakage with exudates 4) retinal ischemia, and 5) neovascular proliferation. Presumably, there is direct retinal microvascular insult from the radiation.

Risk for radiation-induced retinopathy can usually be ascribed to doses exceeding 20 Gy.[38,39] It has been suggested that pre-existing diabetic retinopathy potentiates the onset of radiation retinopathy.[40] The same holds true for systemic microvascular disease caused by hypertension or prior chemotherapy. No long-term complications were encountered in 28 patients who received 20 Gy per orbit after a mean follow-up of 17 months.[18] In another study with 6/14 subjects developed retinopathy, of whom 4 received 30 Gy, one 23 Gy, but one only 20 Gy.[41] All 8 who did not develop retinopathy had total doses of 21 Gy or less. The Stanford group described 242 patients treated with 20 Gy, none of whom developed radiation retinopathy after median follow-up of either 16 or 34 months.[35,36] On the other hand, in one patient only, transitory blindness has been reported shortly after radiotherapy with 20 Gy,[42] and retinopathy has occurred after safe doses as low as 11 Gy and 12 Gy.[43,44] Thus, retinopathy may be a complication of orbital radiotherapy, even at radiation levels previously thought to be safe.

To determine the risk of radiation retinopathy after 20 Gy retrobulbar radiotherapy, 95 ophthalmopathy patients treated between 1982 and 1990, aged 60±13 yr. were recently examined by Tan *et al.*[34] Median time to follow-up was 10 yr. (8-16 yr.). Visual acuity was 0.83±0.24. Nine patients were diabetics, 37 had hypertension. Study parameters were visual acuity, blood pressure, HBA1c, random glucose and a 50° red-free fundus photography with masked grading by 2 observers.

Table 2. Prevalence of retinal changes in patients with Graves' ophthalmopathy (GO): The Amsterdam Graves follow-up Study (contributed by H.S. Tan).[34]

	Proliferative retinopathy	Micro-aneurysms >5	Micro-aneurysms <5	Total	%
GO	0	0	7	7/49	14
GO + hypertension	0	2	4	6/37	16
GO + diabetes	2	1	1	4/9	44

Four of nine patients with diabetes, and 6 of 37 hypertensive subjects showed a retinal changes, and 7 (6 females) of 49 (95% CI: 4.5-24%) non diabetic, non-hypertensive patients had retinal changes (Table 2). No symptomatic retinopathy had occurred at 8-16 yr. after 20 Gy radiotherapy in nondiabetic patients. The mild changes encountered in some of these subjects did not differ in aspect from those encountered in a healthy, nondiabetic population.

Medical applications of ionizing radiation carry the risk of late deterministic and stochastic effects. In general, the dose distribution in the body will be inhomogeneous and the exposed organs have different susceptibilities for tumor induction. The risk of radiation carcinogenesis can be assessed by deriving an effective dose for a standard patient on the basis of the tissue-weighting factors.[45] The attributable life-time risk from small doses is considerably larger at a younger age than later in life (fig. 6). Recently, Snijders-Keilholtz et al.[46] looked at the potential risk of secondary radiation induced malignancies.[47] They suggested that this treatment be reserved for patients above the age of 40-50 yr., because of a risk of fatal secondary cancer of 0.5-0.6% or a cancer incidence of 1.0-1.2% for the irradiation geometry at their hospital and a dose of 20 Gy in the target volume.

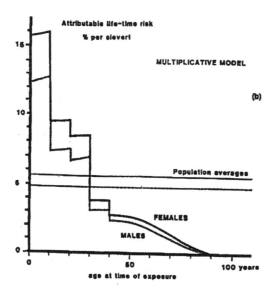

Figure 6. Attributable life time risk of radiation carcinogenesis from a single small dose at various ages at time of exposure assuming a dose, dose rate effectiveness factor (DDREF) of two.[45]

In contrast, Blank *et al.*[48] think that the recommendations of the International Commission on Radiological Protections of 1990 are likely to lead to a 2-4 fold overestimation of the risk. Also, a theoretical risk of 0.3% only, instead of 1.2%, is more appropriate and should be weighted against, (a) complications of alternative treatments, and (b) lifetime cancer risk of about 50% in the general population. In summary, the risk factor for induction of fatal malignancies after retrobulbar radiotherapy can vary between 0.1 and 0.7% and the risk for tumor induction between 0.2 and 1.4%. Since radiation induced malignancies have latency periods of decades the risk for the elderly patient might be limited.

7.   CELL BIOLOGICAL, IMMUNOLOGICAL AND MOLECULAR MECHANISMS

Several questions remain about the use of radiotherapy in Graves' ophthalmopathy, not the least of which is, why does it work? Local immunosuppression is attractive theoretically and was the initial impetus for the trial of this modality. If an aberrant, systemic immune response is the basis of the disease process, it is surprising that symptomatic recurrence is not more common. Possibly radiotherapy interferes with a target other than inflammatory cells, such as the fibroblast or muscle membrane components, to prevent the development of infiltrative changes.[49,50] Radiotherapy takes advantage of the radiosensitivity of the cell mix of orbital tissues in ophthalmopathy. Radiosensitivity of a cell population increases with (a) the ratio of nuclear chromatin to cell mass, (b) the mitotic potential of the cell, and (c) the degree of de-differentiation. Lymphocytes have a high index in all categories and therefore are the most exquisitely sensitive cell line.[51] Lymphocyte reproductive death occurs with doses below 1 Gy and doses greater than 1 Gy induce interphase death. Orbital fibroblasts, possessing a low degree of differentiation and a high proliferative potential, are intermediate on the scale of sensitivity to ionizing radiation, and are sensitive to low dose radiotherapy. At the other end of the spectrum, the most radioresistant cells are those that are highly differentiated and have lost the ability to divide, referred to as fixed postmitotic cells. Included in this class are both striated muscle and neural tissue. Thus, retrobulbar radiotherapy appears to be effective by killing orbital lymphocytes and fibroblasts; consequently retrobulbar radiotherapy might suppress both the mediators (lymphocytes) and the effectors (fibroblasts) of the inflammatory reaction in the orbit.

Ionizing radiation has also been shown to induce a premature terminal differentiation in the fibroblast/fibrocyte cell system.[52,53] In various experimental studies, it could be demonstrated that ionizing radiotherapy (1-10 Gy) induces the terminal differentiation of progenitor fibroblast populations, which are predominantly composed of mitotic fibroblasts, into post-mitotic fibrocytes. This procedure usually requires at least 25-35 cell division cycles. Ionizing radiotherapy, however, induces the post-mitotic fibrocytes within a period of 2-3 weeks, representing approximately 3-4 cell cycles of differentiation divisions. The post-mitotic life span of the fibrocytes experimentally induced by radiotherapy is approximately 40-45% shorter than the life span of post-mitotic fibrocytes arising in normal development of the fibroblast/fibrocyte cell system. For the radiation-induced post-mitotic fibrocytes, it could be demonstrated that the synthesis of interstitial collagen is enhanced by a factor of 5-8.[54] Further, in response to irradiation, resident or recruited macrophages will be stimulated to produce growth factors e.g. specific cytokines like TGF-ß1[55,56] that are capable of expanding the existing fibroblast population[57] or increasing the level of synthesis of extracellular matrix proteins e.g. proteoglycans. Thus, irradiation dramatically alters the ability of macrophages to stimulate normal fibroblast populations, and fibrosis induced by radiation is a multicellular event in which the macrophage and fibroblast cell system interacts through intracellular communication mediated by specific growth factors, especially TGF-ß1.[58,59]

IL-1 has the capacity to stimulate cell proliferation, glycosaminoglycan synthesis and prostaglandin production, and to induce the expression of various immunomodulatory proteins in orbital fibroblasts. It thus has a prominent role in the evolution of the ophthalmopathy. Exposure of orbital fibroblasts to low doses of ultraviolet irradiation enhances their capacity to produce and release IL-1RA. Furthermore, confluent orbital fibroblast monolayers were exposed to increasing doses of irradiation (5 MeV linear accelerator, 0.2-2 Gy), respectively.[60] As demonstrated by RT-PCR and southern hybridization using digoxigenin-labeled oligonucleotide probes specific for the alternate IL-1RA gene variants, irradiation dose-dependently upregulated IL-1RA specific transcripts in ophthalmopathy and control orbital fibroblasts. Further, analysis of IL-1RA protein expression by ELISA revealed enhancement of sIL-1RA expression in culture supernatant of ophthalmopathy and control orbital fibroblasts following irradiation. Thus, therapeutically relevant doses of irradiation act to modulate the expression of IL-1RA gene and protein variants in human orbital fibroblasts. Stimulation of local IL-1RA expression in target cells of the orbital immune process may represent an important mechanism by which orbital radiotherapy exerts its beneficial therapeutic actions in patients with active ophthalmopathy.

8.   CONCLUSIONS

As reviewed, several studies have indicated the efficacy of radiotherapy, which putatively rests on the radiosensitivity of lymphocytes infiltrating the orbit as well as on the reduced proliferation and production of glycosaminoglycans by orbital fibroblasts. The most remarkable improvements occur in eye disease of recent onset (or with recent aggravation). The effects are most notable on the soft tissue changes, and the eye muscle motility disturbances, whereas proptosis is usually unaffected. However, at least one third of the irradiated patients will still require post-treatment corrective eye surgery.

In the era of evidence-based medicine, the use of orbital radiotherapy in patients with ophthalmopathy should be firmly based on prospective randomized trials using validated end-points and strict follow-up. Because only potential improvement but not cure is observed and because the patients themselves are not always satisfied with the results, additional impeccably controlled studies are required. In skilled hands, orbital radiotherapy may be regarded as almost safe and probably effective, particularly in patients with disease of recent onset or brief duration. Using modern techniques, smaller fields, lower and protracted fractionated doses, the risk of secondary tumors, especially in the older age group, might be less than previously estimated and the risks of radiotherapy must be balanced against the risks of alternative treatment which are also not negligible. Until we know more about the long term efficacy, safety (updating of risk estimates by calculation of the total effective dose), required necessary fraction dose and optimal application form, we actually cannot consider orbital radiotherapy as a generally accepted and definitively established treatment. The indications for retrobulbar radiotherapy (clinically active eye disease and prominent inflammatory soft tissue signs, recent onset of progressive proptosis, subacute or acute ophthalmoplegia) remain acceptable until the availability of more definitive results dictate otherwise.

9.   REFERENCES

1. Leer JWH, van Houtte P, Davelaar J. Indications and treatment schedules for irradiation of benign diseases: a survey. Radiother Oncol 1998; 48: 249-257
2. Juler FA. Acute purulent keratitis in exophthalmic goiter treated by repeated tarsorrhaphy resection of cervical sympathetis and x-rays: retention of vision in one eye. Trans Ophthalmol Soc UK 1913; 33: 58-62
3. Mandeville FB. Roetgen therapy of orbital-pituitary portals for progressive exophthalmos following subtotal thyroidectomy. Radiology 1943; 41: 268-271

4. Jones A. Orbital x-ray therapy of progressive exophthalmos. Br J Radiol 1951; 24: 637-646

5. Beierwaltes WH. X-ray treatment of malignant exophthalmos: a report of 28 patients. J Clin Endocrinol 1953; 13: 1090-1100

6. Bahn RS, Heufelder AE. Pathogenesis of Graves'ophthalmopathy. N Engl J Med 1993; 329: 1468-1475

7. Burch HB, Wartofsky L. Graves'ophthalmopathy: current concepts regarding pathogenesis and management. Endocrin Rev 1993; 14: 747-93

8. Kahaly G, Hansen C, Felke B, Dienes HP. Immunohistochemical staining of retrobulbar adipose tissue in Graves'ophthalmopathy. Clin Immunol Immunopathol 1994; 73: 53-62

9. Otto E, Ochs K, Hansen C, Wall J, Kahaly G. Orbital tissue-derived T lymphocytes from patients with Graves'ophthalmopathy recognize autologous orbital antigens. J Clin Endocrinol Metab 1996; 81: 3045-3050

10. Förster G, Otto E, Hansen C, Ochs K, Kahaly GJ. Analysis of orbital T cells in Thyroid-Associated Opthalmopathy. Clin Exp Immunol 1998; 112: 427-434

11. Hansen C, Fraiture B, Rouhi R, Otto E, Förster G, Kahaly G. HPLC glycosaminoglycan analysis in patients with Graves'disease. Clin Science 1997; 92: 511-517

12. Hansen C, Rouhi R, Förster G, Kahaly GJ. Increased Sulfatation of Orbital Glycosaminoglycans in Graves' Ophthalmopathy. J Clin Endocrinol Metab 1999; 84:1409-1413.

13. DeGroot LJ, Gorman CA, Pinchera A, *et al.* Radiation and Graves' ophthalmopathy. Therapeutic controversies. J Clin Endocrinol Metab 1995; 80: 339-349

14. Bartalena L, Marcocci C, Manetti L, *et al.* Orbital radiotherapy for Graves' ophthalmopathy. Thyroid 1998; 8: 439-441

15. Marcocci C, Bartalena L, Bruno-Bossio G, *et al.* Orbital radiotherapy in the treatment of endocrine ophthalmopathy: Why and when? In: Kahaly G (ed) Endocrine Ophthalmopathy – Molecular, immunological and clinical aspects. Karger, Basel, 1993: 131-141

16. Sautter-Bihl M-L. Orbital radiotherapy: recent experience in Europe. In: Wall JR, How J, eds. Graves' ophthalmopathy. Cambridge: Blackwell 1990; 145-157

17. Wiersinga WM, Smit T, Schuster-Uittenhoeve ALJ, van der Gaag, Koornneef L. Therapeutic outcome of prednisone medication and of orbital irradiation in patients with Graves' ophthalmopathy. Ophthalmologica 1988; 197: 75-84

18. Olivotto IA, Ludgate CM, Allen LH, Rootman J. Supervoltage radiotherapy for Graves' ophthalmopathy. CCABC technique and results. Int J Radiation Oncol Biol Phys 1985; 11: 2085-2090

19. Sandler HM, Rubenstein JH, Fowble BL, Sergott RC, Savino PJ, Bosley TM. Results of radiotherapy for thyroid ophthalmopathy. Int J Radiat Oncol Biol Phys 1989; 17: 823-827

20. Kao SCS, Kendler DL, Nugent RA, Adler JS, Rootman J. Radiotherapy in the management of thyroid orbitopathy. Arch Ophthalmol 1993; 111: 819-823

21. Nakahara H, Noguchi S, Murakami N, *et al.* Graves'ophthalmopathy: MR evaluation of 10-Gy versus 24-Gy irradiation combined with systemic corticosteroids. Radiology 1995; 196: 857-862

22. Prummel MF, Wiersinga WM, Mourits MP, Koorneef L, Berghout A, vd Gaag R. Influence of abnormal thyroid function on the severity of accompanying Graves' ophthalmopathy. Arch Int Med 1990; 150: 1098-1101

23. Erickson BA, Harris GJ, Lewandowski MF, Murray KJ, Massaro BM. Echographic monitoring of response of extraocular muscles to irradiation in Graves' ophthalmopathy. Int J Radiat Oncol Biol Phys 1995; 31: 651-660

24.Prummel MF, Mourits MP, Blank L, Berghout A, Koorneef L, Wiersinga WM. Randomised double-blind trial of prednisone versus radiotherapy in Graves' ophthalmopathy. Lancet 1993; 342: 949-954

25.Mourits MP. Randomized double blind trial of orbital radiotherapy vs sham irradiation in Graves'ophthalmopathy. VIth International Symposium on Graves'ophthalmopathy, Amsterdam, NL, Nov. 27-28, 1998

26.Gorman CA. Orbital radiotherapy for Graves'opthalmopathy: a randomized, double blind, prospective, clinical trial. VIth International Symposium on Graves'ophthalmopathy, Amsterdam, NL, Nov. 27-28, 1998

27.Hildebrandt G, Seed MP, Freemantle CN, Alam CAS, Colville-Nash PR, Trott KR. Mechanisms of the anti-inflammatory activity of low-dose radiation therapy. Int J Radiat Biol 1998; 74:367-378

28.Kahaly GJ. Low vs high dose radiotherapy for Graves'opthalmopathy. VIth International Symposium on Graves'ophthalmopathy, Amsterdam, NL, Nov. 27-28, 1998

29.Ravin JG, Sisson JC, Knapp WT. Orbital radiation for the ocular changes of Graves'disease. Am J Ophthalmol 1975; 79: 285-288

30.Trott KR. Therapeutic effects of low radiation doses. Strahlenther Onkologie 1994; 170: 1-12

31.McCartney-Francis N, Allen JB, Mizel DE, *et al.* Suppression of arthritis by an inhibitor of nitric oxide synthase. J Exp Med 1993; 178: 749-754

32.Hofbauer LC, Mühlberg T, Konig A, Heufelder G, Schworn HD, Heufelder AE. Soluble Interleukin-1 receptor antagonist serum levels in smokers and nonsmokers with Graves' ophthalmopathy undergoing orbital radiotherapy. J Clin Endocrinol Metab 1997; 82: 2244-2247

33.Bartalena L, Marcocci C, Tanda ML, *et al.* Cigarette smoking and Graves' ophthalmopathy. Ann Intern Med 1998; 129: 632-635.

34.Tan HS. Orbital radiotherapy in Graves'ophthalmopathy: is it safe? VIth International Symposium on Graves'ophthalmopathy, Amsterdam, NL, Nov. 27-28, 1998

35.Kriss JP, Petersen IA, Donaldson SS, McDougall IR. Supervoltage orbital radiotherapy for progressive Graves'opthalmopathy: results of a twenty year experience. Acta Endocrinol 1989; 121: 154-159

36.Petersen IA, Kriss JP, McDougall IR, Donaldson SS. Prognostic factors in the radiotherapy of Graves'ophthalmopathy. Int J Radiat Oncol Biol Phys 1990; 19: 259-264

37.Miller ML, Goldberg SH, Bullock JD. Radiation retinopathy after standard radiotherapy for thyroid-related ophthalmopathy. Am J Ophthalmol 1991; 112: 600-601

38.Kinyoun JL, Kalina RE, Brower SA, Mills RP, Johnson RH. Radiation retinopathy after orbital irradiation for Graves'ophthalmopathy. Arch Ophthalmol 1984; 102: 1473-1476

39.Parker RG, Withers HR. Radiation retinopathy. JAMA 1988; 259: 43

40.Viebahn M, Marricks ME, Osterloh MD. Synergism between diabetic and radiation retinopathy: case report and review. Br J Ophthalmol 1991; 75: 29-32

41.Nikoskelainen E, Joensuu H. Retinopathy after irradiation for Graves'ophthalmopathy. Lancet 1989; 2: 690

42.Nygaard B, Specht L. Transitory blindness after retrobulbar irradiation of Graves' ophthalmopathy. Lancet 1998; 351: 725-726

43.Elsas T, Thorud E, Jetne V, Conradi IS. Retinopathy after low dose irradiation for an intracranial tumor of the frontal lobe. Acta Ophthalmol 1988; 66: 65-68

44.Lopez PF, Sternberg P, Dabbs CK, Volgler WR, Crocker I, Kalin NS. Bone marrow transplant retinopathy. Am J Ophthalmol 1991; 112: 635-646

45.Broerse JJ. Calculation of effective dose for irradiation of Graves'ophthalmopathy. VIth International Symposium on Graves'ophthalmopathy, Amsterdam, NL, Nov. 27-28, 1998

46.Snijders-Keilholz A, De Keizer RJ, Goslings BM, Van Dam EWCM, Jansen JThM, Broerse JJ. Probable risk of tumour induction after retroorbital irradiation for Graves'ophthalmopathy. Radiother Oncol 1996; 38: 69-71

47.Van Leeuwen FE, Klokman WJ, Hagenbeek A *et al.* Second cancer risk following Hodgkin's disease: a 20-year follow-up study. J Clin Oncol 1994; 12: 312-325

48.Blank LECM, Barendsen GW, Prummel MF, Stalpers L, Wiersinga W, Koornneef L. Probable risk of tumor induction after retroorbital irradiation for Graves'ophthalmopathy. Radiother Oncol 1996; 40: 187-188

49.Kal HB. Orbital radiotherapy in Graves'ophthalmopathy: is it effective? VIth International Symposium on Graves'ophthalmopathy, Amsterdam, NL, Nov. 27-28, 1998

50.Hendry JH. Biological response modifiers and normal tissue injury after irradiation. Radiat Oncol 1994; 4: 123-132

51.Woloschak GE, Chang-Liu CM. Differential modulation of specific gene expression following high- and low radiations. Radiat Res 1990; 124: 183-187

52.Rodemann HP, Peterson HP, Schwenke K, von Wangenheim KH. Terminal differentiation of human fibroblasts is induced by radiation. Scan Microsc 1992; 5: 1135-1143

53.Rodemann HP, Bamberg M. Cellular basis of radiation-induced fibrosis. Radiother Oncol 1995; 35: 83-90

54.Remy J, Wegrowski J, Crechet F, Martin M, Daburon F. Longterm overproduction of collagen in radiation-induced fibrosis. Radiat Res 1991; 125: 14-19

55.Canney PA, Dean St. Transforming growth factor beta. A promoter of late connective tissue injury following radiotherapy? Br J Radiol 1990; 63: 620-623

56.Martin M, Lefaix JL, Pinton P, Crechet F, Daburon F. Temporal modulation of TGF-ß1 and ß-actin gene expression in pig skin and muscular fibrosis after ionizing radiation. Radiat Res 1993; 134: 63-70

57.Haimovitzfriedemann A, Vlodavsky I, Chaudhuri A, Witte L, Fuks Z. Autocrine effects of fibroblast growth factor in repair of radiation damage in endothelial cells. Cancer Res 1991; 51: 2552-2558

58.Strieter RM, Wiggings R, Phan SH. *et al.* Monocyte chemotactic protein gene expression by cytokine-treated human fibroblasts and the epithelial cells. Biochem Biophys Res Commun 1989; 162: 694-700

59.Langberg CW, Hauer-Jensen M, Sung SS, Kane C. Expression of fibrogenic cytokines in rat small intestine after fractionated irradiation. Radiother Oncol 1994; 32: 29-36

60.Mühlberg T, Spitzweg C, Heberling HJ, Heufelder AE. Regulation of Interleukin-1 receptor antagonist gene and protein variants by radiotherapy in Graves' retroocular fibroblasts. J Endocrinol Invest 1998; 21 (Suppl to no. 4): 67 (Abstract)

Chapter 9

Surgical management of Graves' ophthalmopathy

Maarten Ph. Mourits,* Geoffry E. Rose, James A. Garrity, Marco Nardi, Guido Matton, Leo Koornneef
Department of Ophthalmology, Orbital Center, University Medical Center Utrecht, The Netherlands

1.   INTRODUCTION

Graves' ophthalmopathy (GO) is an orbital disease characterised by a disproportion of orbital volume and orbital contents, which is due to enlargement of extraocular muscles and/or an increase of orbital fat.[1] Although some expansion of the orbital bony walls will occur in patients with longstanding ophthalmopathy, in general, the orbit cannot compensate for the increased contents and as a result the orbital tissues including the eyeball are pushed outward. Thus, proptosis and swollen eyelids are frequent findings in GO.[2] When the orbital connective tissue system is very tight, proptosis will be relatively mild at the cost of increased intraorbital pressure,[3] deep orbital pain and optic neuropathy. Proptosis can, therefore, be considered as a natural decompression.[4] Proptotic eyes, however, are vulnerable to wind, dust and foreign bodies, and the increased exposure of the cornea, together with a distorted juxtaposition of eyeball and eyelid, leads to discomfort, redness and tearing.

Aside from swelling, fibrosis of orbital tissues is the hallmark of GO. Fibrosis and contracture of the extraocular muscles are the cause of motility impairment. Fibrosis in and around the levator palpebrae and the lower lid retractors causes upper and lower lid retraction, which enhances the corneal exposure. Upper lid retraction is the most common finding in GO.[5]

GO is characterized by subjective (pain), functional (tearing, diplopia, reduced vision) and cosmetic (proptosis, lid retraction and lid swelling) changes (Fig. 1). The last must not be underestimated. Cosmetic changes occur frequently in GO and are a major reason for psychological distress and social isolation,[5,6] hardly responding to medical intervention.[7,8,9]

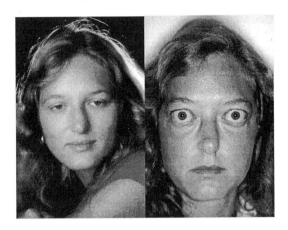

Figure 1. A patient before and after the onset of Graves' ophthalmopathy. Reproduced with permission from the patient.

Sequential surgery aims to correct these anatomical incongruities: Optic nerve compression is relieved by enlarging the bony orbit, which also decreases proptosis; diplopia is reduced by extraocular muscle surgery; eyelid retraction is corrected by lengthening procedures; and, finally, eyelid swelling by blepharoplasty procedures. Optic nerve compression is an urgent problem, in which delay can result in significant visual loss,[10] and patients with optic neuropathy refractive to conservative treatment must undergo orbital decompression immediately. It is common practice to delay all other surgery until euthyroidism and a stable state of ophthalmopathy have been reached. Orbital decompression should precede strabismus surgery, because decompression itself may cause or worsen motility impairment. Eyelid surgery is usually done as a closing procedure, because strabismus surgery (especially on the vertical rectus muscles) may alter lid height position.[11] But all treatment must be tailored to the patient's specific needs.[12] Thus, to camouflage proptosis, one patient might undergo orbital decompression followed by eyelid lengthening, while another patient will be treated with eyelid lengthening alone.

In this chapter, we will describe the various surgical options divided into three subdivisions: decompression surgery, extraocular muscle surgery and eyelid surgery.

2. ORBITAL DECOMPRESSION

2.1 Introduction

Basically, there are three types of surgical orbital decompression in GO:
1. Removal of parts of the bony orbital walls, allowing the orbital contents to expand into the surrounding spaces. 2. Removal of excessive orbital fat. 3. Expansion osteotomies, in which the orbit is put in a more anterior position.

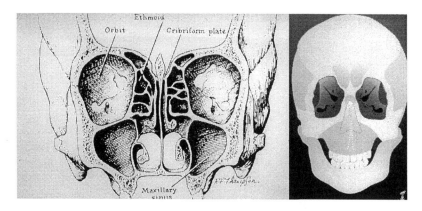

Figure 2. Left panel: Skull showing the thin medial wall and floor that can be removed for decompression; note that the lateral wall is thicker. Right: The grey areas are removed in a three wall decompression (Contributed by M.Ph. Mourits).

Bony wall decompression is the oldest technique: in 1910, Dollinger[13] in Budapest removed the lateral wall of a patient with severe proptosis and corneal ulceration. Today, numerous approaches are applied, of which the most important will be discussed here. One has to realize, however, that orbital decompression is only a first step in functional and cosmetic rehabilitation. Preoperatively, patients must be informed thoroughly about the expected results and the possible complications, especially where orbital decompression is performed for cosmetic reasons only.

2.1.1 Indications

1. impaired visual functions due to optic nerve compression; 2. severe orbital inflammation; 3. reduction of proptosis prior to extraocular muscle surgery; 4. proptosis with severe keratitis; 5. disfiguring proptosis; 6. pain; 7. to alleviate steroid side effects.[14]

In most patients, severe orbital inflammation can be successfully managed with corticosteroids or retrobulbar irradiation. Therefore, orbital decompression is only needed in patients with persistent inflammatory changes refractory to these treatment modalities, or in those in whom the side-effects of these treatments are expected to be worse than a decompression procedure. Keratitis can be successfully managed with local measures such as lubricants, eyelid lengthening or temporary partial tarsorrhaphy. Today, only in patients with severe proptosis and neglected corneal involvement, is a decompression required. Orbital decompression for disfiguring proptosis has been considered too dangerous and was not routinely done before the early 1990's. At that time, however, the surgical procedures had been refined to such a state of perfection that surgeons became confident to decompress orbits for cosmetic reasons only. The term "cosmetic", though, has long been avoided and replaced by rehabilitative.

2.1.2   Preoperative measures

Patients undergoing orbital decompression should be euthyroid and have stable, unchanging ophthalmopathy, unless immediate danger of visual loss is present. Vascular diseases and diabetes mellitus are risk factors, that increase the chance of uncontrollable retrobulbar haemorrhage.[15] Surgery is performed almost always in general anaesthesia. Excessive vomiting and coughing during the immediate postoperative period enhance the risk of retrobulbar bleeding and should be anticipated.

2.1.3   Monitoring

Patients undergoing orbital decompression should be carefully monitored pre- and postoperatively at regular intervals, by assessing corrected visual acuity using a Snellen-chart, exophthalmos with a Hertel exophthalmometer and eyelid aperture with a ruler (including the distance from the upper and lower eyelid border to the corneal limbus), and the presence of lagophthalmos. The amount of eyelid swelling is estimated and photographs are made for comparison.[16] The presence of chemosis (conjunctival edema) and swelling of the caruncle is noted.[17,18] and the cornea inspected with a biomicroscope for punctate keratitis or ulcerations. The optical media are inspected and fundoscopy is performed with special interest for the optic disk or retinal abnormalities (choroidal folds). Ocular pressure is measured in primary position and in elevation. A full orthoptic investigation including presence of binocular single vision and field of binocular single vision, cover test, field of uniocular movements ductions,[19] field of diplopia (if present) and a Hess screen chart is performed. In addition, coronal and axial CT scans are made to assess muscle size, orbital fat mass , bony structures and the state of the paranasal sinuses.

2.1.4 Team approach

To properly manage and evaluate patients with Graves' disease a team consisting of ophthalmologists, endocrinologists and orthoptists is required. Depending on the kind of surgery that will be performed, such a team can be extended with an ENT-surgeon, a plastic surgeon or a neurosurgeon. Some teams work in close cooperation with self-help groups for Graves' patients.

2.2   One-wall decompression techniques

One-wall decompressions are not commonly performed, because reduction of proptosis is generally inadequate. Removal of the floor has been described by Hirsch in 1930,[21] removal of the medial orbital wall by Seawall in 1936,[22] and removal of the lateral wall by Krönlein,[23] which was not originally intended for, but later adapted for GO.[24]

2.3   Two-wall decompression techniques

All sorts of combinations of two-wall decompressions have been described. The removal of the orbital roof, as done by Naffziger in 1931,[25] in fact is a removal of the posterolateral wall. The floor and the medial wall, however, are the structures most frequently removed. They can be reached by a Lynch incision (medial to the eye), by a caruncular incision, by a transconjunctival approach, by a translid, subciliary approach, by a transantral approach and by a transnasal approach.[26] The lateral wall can be removed together with parts of the floor. Some of the techniques will be discussed.

2.3.1   Transantral orbital decompression

The anterior wall of the maxillary sinus is opened through a buccogingival incision and the medial half of the orbital floor and medial orbital wall are removed after the ethmoid air cells have been exenterated. The orbital periosteum is then incised allowing the orbital fat to herniate into the maxillary sinus and into the space created by removal of the ethmoid cells. Naso-anthral windows are placed to allow drainage from the antrum and to prevent post-operative sinusitis. Duration: 90 minutes for both sides.

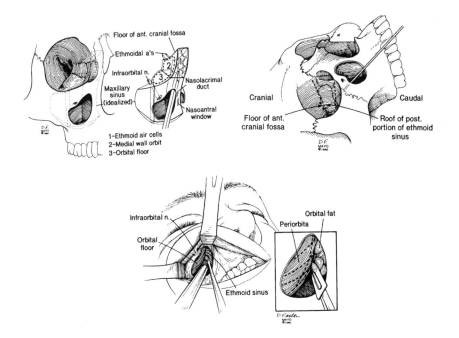

Figure 3. Transantral orbital decompression removes the floor and medial wall of the orbit. Operation begins by opening the maxillary and ethmoid sinuses (upper left). Ethmoidectomy is the most critical portion of the procedure, with a risk for spinal fluid leaks since the roof of the ethmoid sinus is also the floor of the anterior cranial fossa. Note that the posterior portion of the ethmoid roof is located in a more anterior position than the anterior portion of the ethmoid roof (upper right). We recommend that the posterior periorbita be incised in an anterior-posterior direction while the anterior periorbita be incised circumferentially to avoid postoperative diplopia. (Contributed by J.A. Garrity)

2.3.1.1   Results

The transantral approach is one of the most widely used techniques in the world, especially in the USA. Ogura *et al.*[28] reported on the results in 120 patients, Warren *et al.*[29] on 305 patients, Garrity *et al.*[30] on the largest series ever published (namely 428 patients). This last study showed that stabilisation or improvement of visual function was gained in approximately 90%. In patients, in whom the vision did not improve, choroidal folds coursing the macula were often present. The average proptosis reduction was 4.7 mm. The more pronounced the initial proptosis, the greater the degree of proptosis reduction. Long term follow-up studies, show that visual improvement and proptosis reduction are lasting effects.[31,32]

2.3.1.2   Complications

1. Worsening / inducing diplopia (60%), 2. Lower lid entropion (9%), 3. Persistent numb lip (8%), 4. Sinusitis (6%),[33,34] 5. Cerebrospinal fluid leak (4%), 6. Nasolacrimal duct obstruction (3%),[35] 7. Meningitis (< 1%), 8. Loss of vision (< 1%).

2.3.1.3   Comments

The transantral approach is a well established, two-wall decompression technique, in which part of the orbital floor and medial wall are removed. The indications for the surgery, the results and the complications to be expected are well described in literature.[36-40] The operation requires profound knowledge of the anatomy of the skull base, the nose and the paranasal sinuses and for these reasons, the operation is mostly done by ENT-surgeons. The operation has a high rate of increased or induced diplopia.

2.3.2   Translid orbital decompression

A 2.5 cm subciliary incision following the orbitopalpebral skin crease is made. The fibres of the orbicularis muscle are bluntly split and the periosteum covering the lower orbital rim is incised. The periosteum is now elevated from the orbital floor and medial wall. The thin medial part of the floor is perforated and removed as far as the posterior wall of the antral cavity. The nasal orbital wall is removed up to the posterior ethmoidal artery. The sinuses are opened up. The exposed periorbita is incised, enabling the orbital fat to herniate freely into the sinuses. Only the skin is closed. Duration: 40 minutes for both sides.

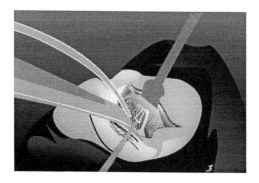

Figure 4. Approach to translid orbital decompression. The infraorbital nerve (white) is clearly visible. (Contributed by M.Ph. Mourits)

2.3.2.1   Results

In the orbital centres of Amsterdam and Utrecht (the Netherlands) several hundreds of translid orbital decompressions have been performed. The reported stabilisation or improvement of vision varied from 70-100%.[41-45] Poor visual recovery after surgery was due to longstanding neuropathy (as indicated by pale disks prior to surgery), choroidal folds or co-existing diabetes mellitus. Proptosis reduction averages 3 mm.

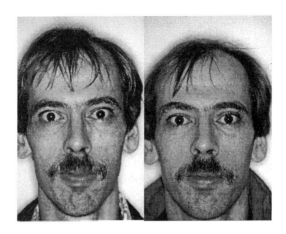

Figure 5. A patient before (left) and 6 months after (right) a translid decompression. Reproduced with permission from the patient. (Contributed by M.Ph. Mourits)

2.3.2.2   Complications

1. Worsening/inducing diplopia (10-20%) 2. Persistent numb lip (5%) 3. Loss of vision (<1%) 4. Inferior displacement of the globe.

2.3.2.3   Comments

The translid approach is also a well-established, two-wall decompression technique and the exposure of the floor is excellent, enabling the infraorbital neurovascular bundle to be respected during surgery. However, the exposure of the medial wall is not as good, which could explain the lesser degree of proptosis reduction in comparison to the transantral decompression. The rate of induced diplopia is low. A translid approach leaves a scar on the eyelid that is hardly visible after some months, except in young individuals (Fig. 5)

2.3.3   'En bloc' resection of the lateral wall and floor

Described by Matton.[46-48] An incision is made in one of the crowfeet and continued subciliarly in the lower eyelid over 1 cm. After elevation of the soft tissues, the periosteum over the lateral wall is incised from the base of the cranium to the zygomatic process and then horizontally over the anterior surface of the maxilla a few millimetres below the orbital rim until the orbital aperture is reached. The periosteum and periorbita are widely undermined and the intraorbital content, the temporalis muscle and the soft tissues over the zygoma are retracted. Using an oscillating saw, the entire lateral wall and the lateral half of the floor with its rim are removed in one piece. Finally, the entire periorbita of the lateral aspect and the lateral part of the floor are excised leaving in place only the anterior lateral strip to which the lateral canthal ligament is attached.

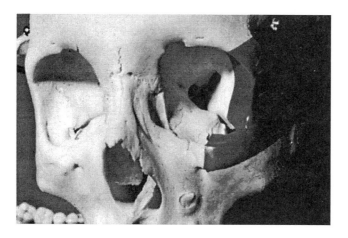

Figure 6. Showing lateral orbital wall and floor to be removed. (Contributed by G. Matton)

2.3.3.1 Results

Matton has used this technique for both patients with optic neuropathy and with disfiguring proptosis. Improvement of vision could be assessed in seven out of ten patients with optic neuropathy. This technique does not allow postoperative measurement using a Hertel exophthalmometer, because resection of the lateral wall makes this measurement inaccurate. However, according to the author, clinical and photographical evaluation showed improvement or complete recovery of disfiguring proptosis in 41/44 patients.

2.3.3.2 Complications

Serious complications were not assessed, Remarkably, diplopia disappeared in four and improved in 12/21 patients with double vision preoperatively, whereas no new diplopia occurred in patients with preoperative normal motility.

2.3.3.3   Comments

So far, the lateral two-wall approach has found few followers. An explanation could be that many surgeons are reluctant to remove parts of the outside of the skull, which are considered to have an important protective function. It has been argued that the temporalis muscle prevents lateral expansion of the orbital content. However, the author has published CT scans, showing expansion of the orbital content and of the lateral rectus muscle into the temporal region.

2.4   Three-wall orbital decompressions

Three-wall decompressions can be considered as extended two-wall decompresssions.[49-51] For instance, Matton in patients with extreme proptosis combined his lateral wall decompression with removal of the part of the floor medial to the infraorbital nerve and even with removal of the medial wall itself. However, some approaches have been specifically developed for three-wall decompression.

2.4.1   Coronal orbital decompression

A skin-muscle incision is made through the scalp 10 mm behind the hair border from tragus (ear) to tragus. The subgaleal flap, including the periosteum, is turned down and the dissection is taken subperiosteal. The superficial temporalis fascia is dissected from the galea and the supraorbital nerves chiselled out of their foramina. The periorbita, including the trochlea, is dissected off the bony walls all around the globe. The temporalis muscle is incised 10 mm from its origin perpendicular to its fibres and the distal part of the muscle is dissected from the bone of the infratemporalis fossa. Periosteum is removed from the zygomaticofrontal process. The lateral wall is removed after coagulation of the frontozygomatic and zygomaticofacial vessels, allowing a fingertip to pass through and leave the rim intact. Medially, after coagulation of the anterior ethmoidal artery, a large part of the lacrimal and ethmoidal bones are removed as far back to the posterior ethmoidal artery. Finally, the floor is perforated and the part medial to the infraorbital nerve and vessels is removed. The periorbita is incised in postero-anterior direction in all quadrants in the posterior part of the orbit and perpendicular to the former in the front.[54] Drains are left behind in the temporalis fossa and removed after 24 hours. The temporalis muscle and fascia is closed with interrupted Vicryl and the skin-muscle flap closed with staples, which are removed after 10 days. Duration: 2 hours.[42,52,53]

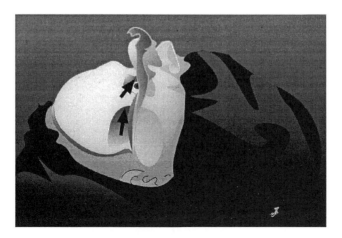

Figure 7. Coronal approach for orbital decompression. The skin flap is turned down and the orbits are approached. (Contributed by M.Ph. Mourits)

2.4.1.1 Results

Stabilisation or improvement is achieved in 80-90% depending on such factors as the preoperative presence of choroidal folds, pale discs, old age and diabetes mellitus, all of which may impair the result. Proptosis reduction ranges from 1 - 14 mm and averages 5 mm.[42-45,55]

2.4.1.2 Complications

1. Numbness of the skin near the scar, 2. Temporal flattening, 3. Worsening of motility impairment (up to 20%). Exceptional complications are: 1. Insufficient proptosis reduction, 2. Too much proptosis reduction requiring orbital wall repair (<1%), 3. Asymmetrical proptosis reduction (e.g. 3 mm or more), 4. Numb lip, 5. Paranasal sinus obstruction, 6. Persistent frontal muscle paralysis, 7. Induced diplopia (up to 10%), 8. Loss of vision (<1%), 9. Cerebrospinal fluid leakage (<1%) and 10. Anosmia (<1%).

2.4.1.3 Comments

The bicoronal approach to the orbits was developed by Tessier to address midfacial fractures and anomalies. Koornneef introduced this technique for decompressions in GO (in Amsterdam) in 1984. The coronal approach enables an optimal exposure and has predictable results. Several hundreds of coronal orbital decompressions have been performed in Amsterdam and Utrecht. The technique has been exported successfully to Belgium, Ireland, Norway, Sweden and finally to Minsk (Belarus), where more than 30 coronals have been performed under difficult surgical circumstances. The advantages of this type of decompression are that it leaves no visible scar and that it can be combined easily with other rehabilitative procedures such as rhytidectomy of the forehead, frontalis and brow lift and with corono-canthopexy. A disadvantage is that this approach is not the preferred approach for baldheaded patients.

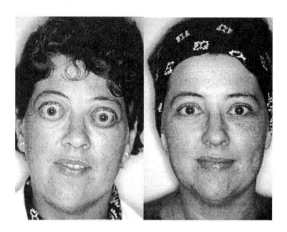

Figure 8. A patient before (left) and 2 weeks after (right) a coronal decompression
Reproduced with permission of the patient. (Contributed by M.Ph. Mourits)

2.4.2   The swinging eyelid decompression

A lateral canthal incision is made, the length of which depends upon the extensiveness of the decompression one wishes to perform. If the lateral wall must be removed, the incision is carried out as far as 1 cm posterior to the posterior edge of the zygomaticofrontal process. Cantholysis of the lower limb of the lateral canthal tendon is performed and the lower lid is everted outward so that an incision can be made through the conjunctiva of the lower fornix. Pulling the eye up, an incision is then made through the capsulopalpebral fascia and orbital fat down to the orbital rim. After elevation of the periorbita, the orbital floor and medial wall can be perforated and removed in a piecemeal manner, sparing the infraorbital neuro-vascular bundle and the attachment of the inferior oblique muscle. To obtain a better view of the medial wall, an additional, caruncular incision or Lynch incision may be made, although this is rarely necessary. The periorbita is incised and the orbital fat can herniate into the surrounding spaces. Before or after this last procedure, the lateral wall is in part excised. The conjunctiva is closed, the lateral canthal tendon is reattached to the periorbita at the lateral orbital rim in the tubercle.[56-58]

2.4.2.1 Results

The results of this technique are a little difficult to evaluate, because in fact it consists of number of procedures that are performed alone or in combination and, in addition, no large series have as yet been published. However, improvement of vision is to expected to be as good as after other decompression techniques. Lyons[59] reported an average 4 mm (range -1.0 to 10 mm) retrodisplacement in 65 orbits (34 patients). According to Rose,[60] larger recessions (average 6-8 mm) can be achieved.

2.4.2.2 Complications

1. Some infraorbital numbness, 2. Worsening/inducing diplopia, 3. Asymmetry, 4. Temporary tenderness of the scar, 5. Enophthalmos.

2.4.2.3 Comments

The exposure through a lateral canthal and inferior fornix incision, first described by McCord, is gaining popularity.[56] The advantage is that it can be combined with an transconjunctival fat blepharoplasty and that it can be tailored very well to the patient's specific needs. The formation of scar tissue, however, may hamper subsequent lower eyelid lengthening to correct lower lid retraction.

2.5 Four-wall orbital decompressions

2.5.1 Technique

A bicoronal incision is made and the dissection is carried out in the subperiosteal plane in the same way as described for the coronal approach. A burr hole is placed at the pterion just behind the frontal process of the frontal bone. With or without additional burr holes, a triangular piece of frontal bone is removed, leaving the dura intact. The frontal sinuses are entered while removing the bone plate, and the mucosa is exenterated from the sinuses. The frontal lobes are carefully retracted in an extradural plane. The roof and lateral wall of the orbit and the sphenoid wing down to the superior orbital fissure are removed with the aid of high speed drills and rongeurs. Extraperiosteal dissection continues within the orbit and the floor and medial wall are removed. The exposed periorbita is incised to ensure complete decompression. The bone flap is repositioned and secured in place, after which the skin-muscle wound is closed.[61-63] Duration: estimated 3 hours.

2.5.1.1   Results

Improvement of visual acuity has been reported in 80% of the patients with diminished vision. Proptosis reduction varied from 2 to 16 mm with an average of 6 mm.

2.5.1.2   Complications

1.New diplopia, 2. Sinusitis, 3. Partial supra- and infraorbital nerve palsy, 4. Partial frontalis paralysis, 5. Enophthalmos.

2.5.1.3   Comments

Four-wall decompressions are performed by neurosurgeons and only small series have been described. These included patients with very severe ophthalmopathy, in whom other decompression techniques had failed.

2.6   Endoscopic decompressions

These are extensions of the standard endoscopic sinus surgery.[64-66] They are two-wall decompressions, in which the medial part of the orbital floor and medial wall are visualized with the aid of an endoscope and then removed. The entrance is endonasal, transconjunctival or transpalpebral. Similar to other decompressions, the aim is herniation of orbital fat and muscle through openings in the periorbita and the orbital walls into the surrounding spaces. Especially in patients with a crowded orbital apex and consecutive neuropathy, the decompression has to reach far back and in this respect the endoscope can be very useful. Improvements of visual functions so far reported are comparable with other decompression techniques. An average proptosis reduction of 4 to 5 mm is described. Some series show a considerable amount of induced diplopia (as much as 100%). All authors agree that endoscopic orbital decompression requires a steep and long learning curve.

2.7   Orbital decompression by fat removal

Described by Olivari.[67-69] An upper eyelid blepharoplasty incision is made, with removal of surplus skin if required. Pulling the orbicularis muscle fibres aside, the orbital septum is visualized, split and the levator palpebrae is identified. Using careful bipolar diathermy, fat and fibrous septa are gradually resected going deeper into the orbit and avoiding the lacrimal nerve. Generally, the lateral fat pads are removed en bloc. Medially above, the supraorbital nerve and superior oblique muscle are identified before fat is excised. Subsequently, the lower lid is incised subciliary and the septum is opened. The inferolateral quadrant allows for the greatest amount of fat excision. Also, fat between the extraocular muscles is removed. Before suturing the orbicularis muscle, the retrobulbar space is irrigated with neomycin and corticosteroid solution. Per orbit about 6 cc fat (range: 3.5-10 cc) is removed. One side at the time is done. Patients are mobilized the same day.

2.7.1   Results

In over 1000 operations in more than 500 patients during more than 10 years, Olivari had a mean proptosis reduction of 6 mm (range: 0-12 mm), corresponding with the same amount (cc) of fat removal. Only occasionally, patients had impaired vision, which then improved in about 60%. Retrobulbar pressure and headaches disappeared almost completely. Instead of inducing diplopia, Olivari found an improvement of motility in the majority of his patients. In contrast to these results, Trokel *et al.* reported an average proptosis reduction of no more 1.8 mm.[68]

2.7.2   Complications

1. temporary diplopia, 2. temporary supraorbital numbness, 3. chemosis. 4. Peroperative hemorrhages.

2.7.3   Comments

Fat resection to decompress the orbit was first described by Moore in 1920,[70] but Pearl[71] showed that fat resection anterior to the axis of the globe does not cause any reduction of proptosis. Only fat removal from within the extraocular muscle corrects exophthalmos. Patients with mainly enlarged extraocular muscles and minimal increased fat tissue would not be good candidates for this procedure and would have little proptosis reduction. Fat resection is not without hazards and Olivari acknowledges that in spite of his low complication rate this operation demands great accuracy, precise technique and meticulous haemostasis.

2.8   Metanalysis of orbital decompression for GO

The large number of approaches and techniques to decompress a bulgy orbit in patients with GO illustrates that no single one is best. Ophthalmologists prefer a lid- or transconjunctival or coronal approach, otorhinolaryngologists a transantral or transnasal approach with or without an endoscope, plastic surgeons are apt to combine procedures and the neurosurgeon favours a transcranial approach. In the right hands, all techniques have shown good results, but there are differences.

Of the four walls of the orbit, the medial and inferior are surrounded by large well-aerated sinuses, affording a major avenue for substantially enlarging the orbit.[51] Superiorly, the orbital roof is adjacent to the frontal lobe laterally to the temporalis muscle. Hence, the most substantial proptosis reduction from orbital decompression can be achieved by removal of the medial and inferior wall. Most authors agree that the more walls removed the more reduction gained. Besides, the larger the preoperative proptosis, the more globe recession can be expected.[30,55] Incision or excision of the periorbita,[72] allowing the orbital contents to protrude through the osteal openings are the keystones to proptosis reduction, although some degree of herniation of orbital contents can be achieved leaving the periorbita intact, as shown by Harvey[73] in three patients. In contrast, we have seen cases, in which the orbital contents were so much fibrosed, that even after complete destruction of the periorbita, the fat would not protrude.

In terms of vision improvement it seems that the preoperative ocular state, rather than the technique are key to the outcome (as long as the orbital apex is addressed). Organized choroidal folds will not disappear, whatever orbital decompression technique is used, and optic atrophy is irreversible.

As to the rate of worsening or induced diplopia, many authors have claimed that their approach is best. Reviewing the literature, one comes to the conclusion that comparison is impossible for the following reasons:

1. Most series are small (less than 50 patients) making statistical evaluation impossible. In addition, series fall apart in even smaller subgroups.
2. Several authors use different treatments at the same time (e.g. surgery plus steroids). So it is impossible to say what is the effect of the surgery and what of the other treatment(s).
3. In many series, no distinction is made between patients who were euthyroid and who were not, between active and quiescent ophthalmopathy, between operations done because of neuropathy or because of disfigurement.
4. There is no agreement on the time interval of assessment of the operation effect. Is it realistic to attribute proptosis reduction to an operation by itself 6 or 12 months after the surgery, when GO is considered to be a self-limiting disease?
5. There is no agreement on the assessment of motility changes.

Unless we agree on these issues, exact comparison remains impossible. What can be concluded from these studies is that, although improvement of motility is sometimes seen, worsening or inducing diplopia is the most significant side-effect of almost all types of orbital decompression. Esotropia and hyper- or hypotropia are most commonly observed after decompression, especially when a medial wall removal is part of the decompression. Many theories exist on the origin of the impaired motility. McCord[57] with postoperative CT scans showed that the more apically a medial wall is removed, the more proptosis reduction is achieved, the better the improvement of vision, but the more motility impairment. The posterior ethmoids support the medial rectus muscle and their absence is proposed to be related to a higher rate of diplopia. Koornneef and Fells[74] hypothesized that symmetrical incisions of the periorbita in all quadrants, enabling the orbital contents to herniate in all directions, would prevent worsening of diplopia. Some authors recommend to leave a bone strut in floor/medial wall decompression to support the globe and to prevent diplopia, the significance of such a strut has never been tested. Worsening of motility can also be the expression of progressive ophthalmopathy itself and cannot be discriminated from surgical effects when patients are operated in the active stage of the disease. Extended destruction of the periorbita may involve the pulleys of the rectus muscles, recently described by Demer[75] and further dynamic and kinematic studies may cast light on these problems.

What does decompression do to the course of the disease itself? Feldon has pointed at the congestive features of GO, which disappear after surgery.[76] However, others have noticed enlargement of the extraocular muscles after orbital decompression.[77] GO symptoms are related to inflammatory changes and congestion of the orbital contents and in many patients, these cannot be distinguished from each other. It is conceivable, that orbital decompression relieves congestive features, but it less likely that it influences the inflammatory process.

Several studies have evaluated patient satisfaction after orbital decompression with special interest for the cosmetic improvements. It was found that the average satisfaction rate was very high, in spite of complications such as lasting numbness and diplopia (provided that this diplopia could be corrected).[45] It appears, that the psychological effects of proptosis reduction in patients with GO cannot be overestimated.

2.9   References

1. Burch HB, Wartofsky L. Graves' ophthalmopathy: Current concepts regarding pathogenesis and management. Endocrine Review 1993; 14:747-793.
2. Wiersinga WM, Smit T, van der Gaag R, Mourits MP, Koornneef L. Clinical presentation of Graves' ophthalmopathy. Ophthalmic Res 1989; 21:73-82.
3. Koornneef L. Eyelid and orbital fascial attachments and their clinical significance. Eye 1988; 2:130-134.
4. Mourits MP. Management of Graves' ophthalmopathy. Rodopi 1990, Amsterdam, NL

5. Bartley GB. The epidemiologic characteristics and clinical course of ophthalmopathy associated with autoimmune thyroid disease in Olmsted county. Trans Am Ass Ophthalmol 1994; 92:477-588.
6. Gerding MN, Terwee CB, Dekker FW, Koornneef L, Prummel MF, Wiersinga WM. Quality of life in patients with Graves' ophthalmopathy is markedly decreased: Measurements by Medical Outcome Study instrument. Thyroid 1993; 14:747-793.
7. Bahn RS, Gorman CA. Choice of therapy and criteria for assessing treatment outcome in thyroid-associated ophthalmopathy. Endocrinol Metab Clin North Am 1987; 16:391-407.
8. Prummel MF, Mourits MP, Berghout A, *et al.* Prednisone and cyclosporine in the treatment of severe Graves' ophthalmopathy. N Engl J Med 1989; 321:1353-1359.
9. Prummel MF, Mourits MP, Blank L, Koornneef L, Wiersinga WM. Randomised double-blind trial of prednisone versus radiotherapy in Graves' ophthalmopathy. Lancet 1993; 342:949-54.
10. Trobe JD, Glase JS, Laflamme P. Dysthyroid optic neuropathy. Clinical profile and rationale for management. Arch Ophthalmol 1987; 96:1199-1209.
11. Shorr N, Seiff SR. The four stages of surgical rehabilitation of the patient with dysthyroid ophthalmopathy. Ophthalmology 1986; 93:476-483.
12. Hurwitz JJ, Birt D. An individualized approach to orbital decompression in Graves' orbitopathy. Arch Ophthalmol 1985; 103:660-665.
13. Dollinger J. Die Druckenentlastung der Augenhöhle durch Entfernung der äusseren Orbitalwand bei hochgradigem Exophthalmous (Morbus Basedowii) und konsekutiver Hornhauterkrankung. Deutsche Med Wochenschr 1911; 41:1888-1890.
14. DeSanto LW. Transantral orbital decompression. In: Gorman CA, Waller RR, Dyer JA, eds. The eye and orbit in thyroid disease. New York: Raven Press 1984: 231-251.
15. Kalmann R, Mourits MP. Diabetes mellitus; A risk factor in patients with Graves' orbitopathy. Br J Ophthalmol 1999; 83:463-465.
16. Gerding MN, Prummel MF, Kalmann R, Koornneef L, Wiersinga WM. The use of colour slides in the assessment of changes in soft-tissue involvement in Graves' ophtha lmopathy. J Endocrinol Invest 1998; 21:459-462.
17. Mourits MP, Koornneef L, Wiersinga WM, Prummel MF, Berghout A, van der Gaag R. Clinical criteria fir the assessment of disease activity in Graves' ophthalmopathy: a novel approach. Br J Ophthalmol 1989; 73:639-644.
18. Mourits MP, Prummel MF, Wiersinga WM, Koornneef L. Clinical activity score as a guide in the management of patients with Graves' ophthalmopathy. Clin Endocrinol 1997; 47:9-14.
19. Mourits MP, Prummel MF, Wiersinga WM, Koornneef L. Measuring eye movements in Graves' ophthalmopathy. Ophthalmology 1994; 101:1341-1346.
20. Alper MG. Pioneers in the history of orbital decompression for Graves' ophthalmopathy. Doc Ophthalmol 1995; 89:163-71.
21. Hirsch VO, Urbanek I. Behandlung eines excessiven Exophthalmus (Basedow) durch Entfernung von Orbitafett von der Kieferhohle aus. Monatsschr für Ohrenheilk Laryngorhinol 1930; 64:212-3.
22. Sewall EC. Operative control of progressive exophthalmos. Arch Otolaryngol 1936; 24:621-624.
23. Krönlein RU. Zur pathologie und operativen Behandlung der Dermoid-cysten der Orbita. Betr. Klin Chir 1888; 4:149-163.
24. Berke RN. A modified Krönlein operation. Trans Am Ophthalmol Soc 1953; 51:193-231.
25. Naffziger HC. Progressive exophthalmos following thyroidectomy: Its pathology and treatment. Ann Surg 1931; 94:582-586.

26. Rootman J, Stewart B, Goldberg RA, eds. Decompression for thyroid orbitopathy. In: Orbital surgery. A conceptual approach. Lippincott-Raven, Philadelphia 1995, 353-384.

27. Walsh ThE, Ogura JH. Transantral orbital decompression for malignant exophthalmos. Laryngoscope 1957; 67:544-567.

28. Ogura JH, Lucente FE. Surgical results of orbital decompression for malignant exophthalmos. Laryngoscope 1974; 84:637-644.

29. Warren JD, Spector JG, Burde R. Long-term follow-up and recent observations on 305 cases of orbital decompression for dysthyroid orbitopathy. Laryngoscope 1989; 99:35-40.

30. Garrity JA, Fatourechi V, Bergstralh EJ, Bartley GB, Beatty ChW, DeSanto LW, Gorman CA. Results of transantral orbital decompression in 428 patients with severe Graves' ophthalmopathy. Am J Ophthalmol 1993; 116:533-547.

31. Hutchison BM, Kyle PM. Long-term visual outcome following orbital decompression for dysthyroid eye disease. Eye 1995; 9:578-581.

32. Lee AG, McKenzie BA, Miller NR, Loury MC, Kennedy DW. Long term results of orbital decompression in thyroid eye disease. Orbit 1995; 14:59-70.

33. Bough ID, Huang JJ, Pribitkin EA. Orbital decompression for Graves' disease complicated by sinusitis. Ann Otol Rhinol Laryngol 1994; 103:988-990.

34. Lee WC. Recurrent frontal sinusitis complicating orbital decompression in Graves' disease. J Laryngolol Otol 1996; 110:670-672.

35. Seiff SR, Shor N. Nasolacrimal drainage system obstruction after orbital decompression. Am J Ophthalmol 1988; 106:204-209.

36. Tjon F, Knegt P, Eijngaarde R, Poublon R, van der Schans E, Krenning E. Transantral orbital decompression for Graves' disease. Clin Otolaryngol 1994; 19:290-294.

37. Sverker Hallin E, Feldon SE, Luttrell J. Graves' ophthalmopathy: III. Effect of transantral orbital decompression on optic neuropathy. Br J Ophthalmol 1988; 72: 683-687.

38. McNab AA. Orbital decompression for thyroid orbitopathy. Austr N Zealand J Ophthalmol 1997; 25:55-61.

39. Fatourechi V, Garrity JA, Bartley GB, Bergstralh EJ, DeSanto LW, Gorman CA. Graves ophthalmopathy. Results of transantral orbital decompression performed for cosmetic indications. Ophthalmology 1994; 101:938-942.

40. Fatourechi V, Bergstralh, Garrity JA, Bartley GB, Beatty ChW, Offord KP, Gorman CA. Predictors of response to transantral orbital decompression in severe Graves' ophthalmopathy. Mayo Clin Proc 1994; 69:841-848.

41. Härting F, Koornneef L, Peeters HJ, Gillissen PA. Fourteen years of orbital in Graves' disease. Orbit 1986; 5:123-129.

42. Koornneef L, Mourits MP. Orbital decompression for decreased visual acuity or for cosmetic reasons. Orbit 1988; 7:225-238.

43. Mourits MP, Koornneef L, Wiersinga WM, Prummel MF, Berghout A, van der Gaag R. Orbital decompression for GO by inferomedial, by inferomedial plus lateral, and by approach. Ophthalmology 1990; 97:636-641.

44. Versteegh MFL, Mourits MP. Treatment of optic neuropathy and disfiguring proptosis by orbital decompression in patients with Graves' orbitopathy. MEJO 1996.

45. Paridaens D, Hans K, van Buitenen S, Mourits MP. The incidence of diplopia following coronal and translid orbital decompression in Graves' orbitopathy. Eye 1998; 12:800-805.

46. Matton G. Resection "en bloc" of the lateral wall and floor for decompression of the in dysthyroid exophthalmos. Eur J Plast Surg 1991; 14:114-119.

47. Matton G. Recent advances in orbital surgery for exophthalmos. Adv Plast Reconstr 1993; 9:103-125.

48. Matton G. Orbital decompression by "en bloc" resection of the lateral orbital wall and floor. In: Van der Meulen JC, Gruss JS (eds) Color atlas and text of ocular plastic surgery. London: Mosby-Wolfe, 117-122.

49. Wolfe SA. Modified three-wall orbital expansion to correct persistent exophthalmos or exorbitism. Plast Reconstr Surg 1979; 64:448-455.

50. Buschmann W, Richter W, Kruse Ph, Neumann O. Functional results in Graves' disease following ophthalmo-rhinosurgical orbital decompression. Orbit 1986; 5:117-121.

51. Kulwin DR, Cotton RT, Kersten RC. Combined approach to orbital decompression. Otolaryngolol Clin N Am 1990; 23:381-390.

52. Tessier P. Expansion chirurgicale de l'orbite. Ann Chir Plast 1969; 14:207-214.

53. Krastinova D, Rodallec A. Orbitopathie Basedowienne. Ann Chir Plast Esthét 1985; 30:351-358.

54. Koornneef L. Orbital bony and soft tissue anatomy. In: Gorman CA, Waller RR, Dyer JA (eds): The eye and orbit in thyroid disease. New York, Raven Press 1984, 5-23.

55. Kalmann R, Mourits MP, van der Pol JP, Koornneef L. Coronal approach for orbital decompression in GO. Br J Ophthalmol 1997; 81:41-45.

56. McCord CD. Orbital decompression for Graves' disease. Exposure through lateral and inferior fornix incision. Ophthalmology 1981; 88:533-541.

57. McCord CD. Current trends in orbital decompression. Ophthalmology 1985; 92:21-33.

58. Antoszyk JH, Tucker N, Codère F. Orbital decompression for Graves' disease: Exposure through a modified blepharoplasty incision. Ophthalmic Surg 1992; 23:516-521.

59. Lyons ChJ. Rootman J. Orbital decompression for disfiguring exophthalmos in thyroid orbitopathy. Ophthalmology 1994; 101:223-230.

60. Rose G. Personal communication during the VIth International symposium of Graves' ophthalmopathy, Amsterdam, November 27-28, 1998.

61. Kennerdell JS, Maroon JC. An orbital decompression for severe dysthyroid. Ophthalmology 1982; 89:467-472.

62. Stranc M, West M. A four-wall orbital decompression for dysthyroid orbitopathy. J Neurosurg 1988; 68:671-677.

63. West M, Stranc M. Long term results of four-wall orbital decompression for Graves' ophthalmopathy. Br J Plast Surg 1997; 50:507-516.

64. Metson R, Dallow RL, Shore JW. Endoscopic orbital decompression Laryngoscope 1994; 104:951-957.

65. Khan JA, Wagner DV, Tiojanco JK, Hoover LA. Combined transconjunctival and approach for endoscopic orbital apex decompression in Graves' disease. Laryngoscope 1995;105:203-206.

66. Lund VJ, Larkin G, Fells P, Adams G. Orbital decompression for thyroid eye disease: a comparison of external and endoscopic techniques. J Laryngol Otol 1997;111: 1051-1055.

67. Olivari N. Transpalpebral decompression of endocrine ophthalmopathy (Graves' disease) by removal of intraorbital fat: Experience with 147 operations over 5 years. Plast & Reconstr Surg 1991; 87:627-641.

68. Trokel S, Kazim M, Moore S. Orbital fat removal. Decompression for Graves. Ophthalmology 1993; 100:674-682.

69. Adenis JP, Robert PY. Décompression orbitaire selon la technique d'Olivari. J Fr Ophthalmol 1994; 17:686-691.

70. Moore RF. Exophthalmos and limitation of eye movements of Graves' disease. Lancet 1920; 2:701.

71. Pearl RM. Surgical management of volumetric changes in the bony orbit. Ann Plast 1987; 19:349-358.

72. Stanley RS, McCaffrey TV, Offord KP, DeSanto LW. Superior and transantral decompression procedures. Arch Otolaryngol Head Neck Surg 1989; 115:369-373.
73. Harvey JT. Orbital decompression for Graves' disease leaving the periosteum intact. Ophthal Plast Reconstr Surg 1989; 5:199-206.
74. Fells P. Orbital decompression for severe dysthyroid eye disease. Br J Ophthalmol 1987; 71:107-111.
75. Demer Jl, Miller JM, Poukens V, Vinters HV, Glasgow BJ. Evidence for fibromuscular pulleys of the recti extraocular muscles Invest Ophthalmol Vis Sc 1995; 36:1125-1136.
76. Feldon S. Personal communication during the VIth International symposium of Graves' ophthalmopathy, Amsterdam, November 27-28, 1998.
77. Wenz R, Levine M, Putterman A, Bersani Th, Feldman K. Extraocular muscle enlargement after orbital decompression for GO. Ophth Plast Reconstr Surg 1994; 10:33-41.

3. EXTRAOCULAR MUSCLE SURGERY

3.1 Introduction

Aside from reduced vision, impaired motility is the most disturbing symptom of GO. It restrains patients from daily private and professional activities and can be the reason why they have to temporarily stop or permanently cease employment. GO is the most frequent cause of 'spontaneous' double vision in middle-age and early senescence, but the reported prevalence of motility impairment in GO varies widely. Limitation of ocular ductions are found in 15 - 70% of patients with GO. [1-4]

Impaired motility is seen frequently in patients with only mild proptosis and some authors consider restrictive myopathy as a distinct subtype of GO, in which fibrotic changes play a more dominant role than in 'proptotic' GO. Graves' myopathy must be differentiated from myasthenia gravis, paralytic strabismus and orbital myositis by orthoptic evaluation and CT-scanning.

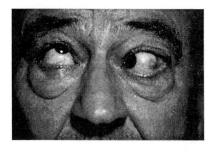

Figure 11. Graves' ophthalmopathy patient with mild proptosis and hypertropia plus esotropia. (Contributed by M.Ph. Mourits)

Diplopia can only develop in individuals with pre-existent binocular single vision and Graves' patients with profound amblyopia or markedly reduced visual acuity of one eye will be 'spared' from diplopia. Limitation of duction does not necessarily cause double vision. Patients with symmetrical limitation of elevation avoid diplopia by raising their chin and complain about neck stiffness and pain instead of diplopia. Many patients are troubled by diplopia in the first hours after awakening, whereas others experience diplopia when they get fatigued. Diplopia may be present only at the extremes of gaze, or may occur in primary and reading position, and a number of patients have the impression that their eyes need more time to follow and get sharp changing objects. It would appear that the regulatory system for ocular ductions is affected first and frank diplopia, if it occurs, follows later. Paradoxically, worsening of the ophthalmopathy sometimes results in less diplopia, as, for example, in patients with unilateral reduced elevation, who later develop bilateral disease.This phenomenon has lead to much misunderstanding at the evaluation of GO, especially among non-ophthalmologists.

The mechanism of impaired motility was not immediately understood. First, it was attributed to paralysis of the muscle at the side of the globe at which the duction was impaired.[5,6] Later, it became clear that it is not so much paralysis, but fibrosis, of the antagonist, which reduces the compliance of the muscle, and thereby reduces motility.[7]

3.2   Patterns of motility disturbance

For reasons not understood, the inferior rectus muscle is involved most frequently, followed in frequency by the medial rectus and superior rectus muscle. The lateral rectus muscle and the oblique muscles are only enlarged in severe forms of orbitopathy.[4,8]

Table 1. Nomenclature of ocular misalignement.

	Ocular misalignement
Esotropia	Inward deviation
Exotropia	Outward deviation
Hypotropia	Downward deviation
Hypertropia	Upward deviation

This predilection of diseased muscles determines the pattern of impaired motility, hypotropia and esotropia (or a combination of both), being most commonly seen.[9-11] In fact, the presence of an exotropia may suggest co-existent myasthenia gravis.[12] Exotropia, in- and excyclodeviations have been described as well, but occur incidentally.[2,13-15] A-patterns were noted by

Fells, especially after anterior ethmoidal orbital decompressions.[16] The selective involvement of the inferior rectus muscle is responsible for the frequently encountered phenomenon of increased intraocular pressure in upgaze, the tight muscle blocking the episcleral aqueous outflow on attempted upgaze.[17-19]

3.3 Motility changes after orbital decompression

De novo origin or aggravation of existent motility impairment is the most common side-effect of almost all sorts of orbital decompression (except in the "en bloc" decompression) with a prevalence varying from 0 to 100% (Table 2).

Table 2. Prevalence of de novo development or worsening of motility disturbances after different methods of orbital decompression surgery for severe optic neuropathy (on), or for rehabilitative (rehab) reasons

Author	Method	Indication	Number of patients	Induced motility abnormalities %
Linberg [47]	Translid	On	9	30
McCord [48]	Swinging eyelid	On + Rehab	34	?
McCord [49]	Translid	On + Rehab	239	6
	Transantral	On + Rehab	159	41
Hurwitz [50]	Transantral	On + Rehab	19	84
	Combined	On + Rehab	40	80-100
Fells [16]	Anterior ethmoidect	On + Rehab	14	79
Mourits [11]	Translid	On + Rehab	27	7
	Coronal	On + Rehab	23	9
Leatherbarow [51]	Coronal	On + Rehab	10	60
Kao [52]	Transantral	On + Rehab	4	75
	Subciliar	On + Rehab	13	54
	Transfornical	On + Rehab	6	17
Garrity [53]	Transantral	On + Rehab	428	64
Fatourechi [54]	Transantral	Rehab	34	73
Lyons [55]	?	Rehab	34	29
Kalmann [56]	Coronal	Rehab	125	22
Paridaens [57]	Translid	On	6	33
		Rehab	29	14
	Coronal	On	5	20
		Rehab	41	20

The occurrence of diplopia after orbital decompression is, however, less remarkable than its absence. During most orbital decompressions not only are large parts of the orbital walls removed, but also parts of the periorbita, to which the suspensory fibrous connective tissue skeleton of the orbit is attached.[20] For instance, in coronal orbital decompression the trochlea is completely detached from its fastening to the orbital roof, yet, postoperative weakening of the superior oblique muscle is rarely observed. Removal of the medial wall and floor cause a medial and downward displacement of the orbital contents, pulling the extraocular muscles in different planes, but the effect on functional anatomy of the rectus muscles has not been clarified. Adhesions resulting from intraorbital haemorrhage during surgery could cause motility impairment, just as in orbital fractures. For these reasons, it is intriguing to question why not all patients develop double vision after decompression. Obviously, some self-regulatory system (orthophorization) is involved and Huber found that GO-patients develop an abnormally large fusion range, especially in the vertical plane.[21]

Some investigators believe that orbital decompression predispose a patient to a higher risk of reoperation, but if this is caused by the decompressive procedure itself or by the fact that candidates for orbital decompression suffer from more advanced orbitopathy remains to be concluded. Nunery *et al.*,[22] divided GO-patients in two categories: Type 1 patients have normal versions and will only occasionaly develop diplopia after decompression, whereas type 2 patients (those with restrictive motility loss and diplopia within 200 of the primary position) are most likely to develop diplopia after decompressive surgery.

3.4   Non-surgical treatment for diplopia

Patients with diplopia and a constant, but not too large an angle of strabismus can be helped with prisms. When the angle is still changing and if Fresnel prisms are not satisfactory, then temporary occlusion of one eye, may be indicated. During the early stage of the ophthalmopathy, when 'inflammatory spasm' rather than contracture would be the cause of restriction, motility changes are still reversible, and indeed, spontaneous improvement of motility and abating of diplopia are not uncommon. Improvement of motility is also seen after immunosuppressive treatments or after retrobulbar irradiation.[23,24] In selected cases, temporary improvement can be achieved with Botulinum toxin injections,[25,26] allowing the patient to remain binocular during the acute phase of the disease until stabilisation of signs has been achieved and surgery can be performed.[27]

3.5   Surgical treatment for diplopia

General agreement exists as to the timing of strabismus surgery. The motility pattern should be unchanged for at least 3-6 months. Decompressive surgery, if planned, should be performed prior to squint surgery, as it influences the position and function of the extraocular muscle system. In addition, strabismus surgery without previous decompression in patients with Hertel readings over 23 mm, is said to enhance the risk of corneal involvement.[28]

Binocular single vision in all directions is seldomly achieved. The goal of surgery is, therefore, to achieve binocular single vision in primary and reading positions. Multiple operations and redo-operations may be required to reach that goal. Table 3 supplies a literature overview of the results of squint surgery in patients with GO, the techniques used and the several definitions of success.[1,7,11,29,38]

Table 3. Results of strabismus surgery in ophthalmopathy. Success is defined either according to fusion in primary position (PP), in reading position (RP), or to binocular single vision (BSV). Results are given according to the use of fixed (fix) sutures, or adjustable (adj) sutures.

Author	Nr of patients	Technique	Definition of success	Success rate (%)	Overcorrec- tion (%)
Miller[7]	7	Recession, fix	PP + RP	72	0
Ellis[14]	30	Recession, adj	"Good results"	83	0
Scott[1]	22	Recession, adj	PP	82	18
Evans[2]	45	Recession, fix	PP + RP	65 (PP), 57 (RP)	9
Sterk[29]	20	Recession, resection, fix	PP + RP	70	0
Mailette[13]	22	Recession, fix	PP + RP	73	0
Fells[36]	32	fix	PP + RP	66	
	38	Adj	PP + RP	76	
Gardner[30]	30	Recession, adj	Orthophoric	95	
Mourits[11]	38	Recession, resection, fix	PP + RP	71	
Fells[37]	58	Recession, adj	PP + RP	60	
Lueder[33]	58	Recession, adj	PP + RP	47	
Kraus[35]	26	Recession, fix	PP + RP	38	31
	11	Recession, adj	PP + RP	64	28
Nardi[46]	20	Tendon lengthening	?	?	15
Fells[38]	41	Recession, adj	BSV	49	24

Weakening of the restricted muscle is the operation of choice, either in the form of a recession, with fixed or with adjustable sutures, or in the form of a lengthening procedure. Using adjustable sutures, a double-armed 6.0 Vicryl suture is brought through a long scleral tunnel starting posterior to the original muscle insertion and ending just anterior to it. After severing from its insertion, the muscle is placed in the appropriate position and temporarily tied down in an adjustable knot. Conjunctiva and Tenon's capsule are recessed to eliminate any restrictive effect they may have. Six to 24 hour after the operation, using topical anaesthesia, the suture is adjusted and definitively tied.[39] Resections are performed only occasionally. Success rates vary from 38% in the patients operated with fixed sutures in the study of Kraus,[35] to 95% in Gardner's study on adjustable sutures.[30] Comparing the use of fixed and adjustable sutures, the latter seem to give better results, especially in the studies of Fells and Kraus,[36-38] who used both techniques. On the other hand, the range of success rate varies more in the adjustable group, possibly illustrating the technical difficulty of the procedure. Recession of the inferior rectus muscle, together with the medial rectus muscle may result in the occurrence of a secondary A-pattern in downgaze, which may be prevented by transposition of the medial muscle upward.

Surgical overcorrection of hypotropia is recognized increasingly as a disagreeable complication, with occurrences up to 31%. Factors contributing to overcorrection seem to be tightness of the ipsilateral superior rectus muscle and tightness of the contralateral inferior rectus muscle, both of which should be examined through the forced duction test during the operation. In addition, in our series, overcorrection was found to occur especially after orbital decompression. Overcorrection in the vertical plane may cause diplopia when reading, which is much more annoying than diplopia in upgaze and therefore should be prevented by aiming at mild undercorrection.

Hudson found a correlation between the amount of proptosis, superior rectus muscle volume and the incidence of overcorrection.[40] Increased volume, however, can cause increased proptosis and tightness of the superior rectus muscle and, therefore, the relation between proptosis and overcorrection seems an indirect one.

Publications on dose-effect ratios in muscle surgery in patients with GO, show results ranging from 1.89 °/mm to 2.1 °/mm for vertical recessions and from 1.75 °/mm to 2.1 °/mm for horizontal recessions.[35,41-44] Most strabismus surgeons agree that larger recessions are required in GO patients than for other types of squint.[45] To extend the muscle recession the use of implants such as allogeneic scleral implants has been reported with controversial results.[39,46] We prefer large recessions by suturing the muscle on a loop.

Aside from over- or undercorrection, increased lower lid retraction is a frequent complication of inferior rectus recession, even after extensive cutting of the lower lid retractors and adhesions between the inferior rectus muscle and the lid muscles.

3.6   References

1. Scott WE, Thalacker JA. Diagnosis and treatment of thyroid myopathy. Ophthalmology 1981; 88:493-498.
2. Evans D. Extraocular muscle surgery for dysthyroid myopathy. Am J Ophthalmol 1983; 95:767-771.
3. Bartley GB. The epidemiologic characteristics and clinical course of ophthalmopathy associated with autoimmune thyroid disease in Olmsted county, Minnesota. Trans Am Ass Ophthalmol 1994; 92:477-588.
4. Wiersinga WM, Smit T, Van der Gaag R, Mourits MP, Koornneef L. Clinical presentation of Graves' ophthalmopathy. Opththalmic Res 1989; 21:73-78.
5. Rundle FF, Wilson CW. Ophthalmoplegia in Graves' Disease. Cli Sci 1944; 51:17-29
6. Goldstein JE. Paresis of superior rectus muscle associated with thyroid dysfunction. Arch ophthalmol 1964; 72:5-8.
7. Miller JE, van Heuven W, Ward R. Surgical correction of hypotropias associated with thyroid dysfunction. Arch Ophthalmol 1965; 74:509-515.
8. Feldon SE, Lee CP, Muramatsu SK, Weiner JM. Quantitative CT of Graves' ophthalmopathy. Arch Ophthalmol 1985; 103:213-215.
9. De Waard R, Koornneef L, Verbeeten B. Motility disturbaces in Graves' ophthalmopathy. Doc Ophthalmol 1983; 56:41-47.
10. Omrod JN. Management of squint in dysthyroid disease. Trans Ophthalmol Soc UK 1981; 101:284-298.
11. Mourits MP, Koornneef L, van Mourik-Noordenbos AM, *et al.* Extraocular muscle surgery for Graves' ophthalmopathy. Br J Ophthalmol 1990; 74:81-83.
12. Vargas ME, Warren FA, Kupersmith MJ. Exotropia as a sifn of myasthenia gravis in dysthyroid ophthalmopathy. Br J Ophthalmol 1993; 77:822-823.
13. Maillette de Buy Wenniger-Prick LJJM, van Mourik-Noordenbos AM,Koornneef L. surgery in patients with Graves' ophthalmopathy. Doc Ophthalmol 1986; 61:219-221.
14. Ellis FD. Strabismus surgery for endocrine ophthalmopathy. Ophthalmology 1979; 86:2059-2063.
15. Nardi M, Bartolomei MP, Pinchera A, Barca L. Misleading signs in inferior rectus restrictive disorders. It J Ophthalmol 1990; 4:91-94.
16. Fells P. Orbital decompression for severe dysthyroid eye disease. Br J Ophthalmol 1987; 71:107-111.
17. Gamblin GT, Harper DG, Galentine P, Buck DR, Chernow B, Eil Cl. Prevalence of increased intraocular pressure in Graves' disease-evidence of frequent subclinical. N Engl J Med 1983; 308:420-424.
18. Kalmann R, Mourits MP. Prevalence and management of elevated intraocular pressure in patients with Graves' orbitopathy. Br J Ophthalmol 1998; 82:754-757.
19. Nardi M, Bartolomei MP, Romani A, Barca L. Intraocular pressure changes in secondary positions of gaze in normal subjects and in restrictive motility disorders. Graefe's Arch Clin Exp ophthalmol 1988, 226:8-10.
20. Koornneef L. Spatial aspects of orbital musculo-fibrous tissue in man. Swets & Zeitlinger Amsterdam 1977.
21. Huber A. Ocular motility in Graves' Disease. Neuroophthalmology1984; 4:227-236.
22. Nunery WR, Nenery CW, Martin RT, Truong TV, Osborn DR. The risk of diplopia following orbital floor and medial wall decompression in subtypes of ophthalmic Graves' disease. Ophthalmic Plast Reconstruct Surg 1997; 13:153-160.

23. Prummel MF, Mourits MP, Blank L, Koornneef L, Wiersinga WM. Randomised double-blind trial of prednisone versus radiotherapy in Graves' ophthalmopathy. Lancet 1993; 342:949-954.

24. Mourits MP.Personal communication during the VIth International symposium of Graves' ophthalmopathy, Amsterdam, November 27,28, 1998.

25. Dunn WJ, Arnold AC, O'Connor PS. Botulinum toxin for the treatment of dysthyroid ocular myopathy. Ophthalmology 1986; 93:470-475.

26. Lyons CJ, Vickers SF, Lee JP. Botulinum toxin therapy in dysthyroid strabismus. Eye 1990; 4:538-540.

27. Gavin MP, Kemp EG, Kirkness CM. Botulinum toxin-A in the management of dysthyroid strabismus. Orbit 1997; 16:127-129.

28. Dyer JA. Ocular muscle surgery. In: Gorman CA, Waller RR, Dyer JA (eds). The eye and orbit in thyroid disease. New York: Raven Press 1984,253-261.

29. Sterk CC, Bierlaagh JJM, de Keizer RJW. Motility disorders in endocrine ophthalmopathy. Doc Ophthalmol 1985; 59:71-75.

30. Gardner TA, Kennerdell JS. Treatment of dysthyroid myopathy with adjustable suture recession. Ophthalmis Surg 1990; 21:519-24.

31. Kolling JH. Experiences with recess/resect procedures on horizontal and vertical rectus muscles in the treatment of Graves' Ophthalmopathy. Trans Europ Strabismol Ass 1991

32. Fishman DR, Benes SC. Upgaze intraocular pressure changes and strabismus in Graves' ophthalmopathy. J Clin Neuroophthalmol 1991; 11:162-165.

33. Lueder GT, Scott WE, Kutschke PJ, Keech RV. Long-term results of adjustable suture surgery for strabismus secondary to thyroid ophthalmopathy. Ophthalmology 1992; 99:993-997.

34. Ohtsuki H, Hasebee S, Kishimoto F. Intraoperative suspension-recession technique for treatment of vertical strabismus in thyroid myopathy. Ophthalmologica 1993; 206:38-44.

35. Kraus DJ, Bullock JD. Treatment of thyroid ocular myopathy with adjustable and nonadjustable suture strabismus surgery. Trans Am Ophthalmol Ass 1993; 91:67-79.

36. Fells P, McCarry B. "Fixed" versus "adjustable" sutures in the treatment of dysthyroid ophthalmopathy. Trans Europ Strabismol Ass 1988.

37. Fells P, McCarry B, Aylward GW. Ocular muscle surgery in thyroid eye disease. Orbit 1992; 11:169-175.

38. Fells P, Kousoulides L, Pappa A, Munro P, Lawson J. Extraocular muscle problems in thyroid eye disease. Eye 1994; 8:497-505.

39. Char DV. Therapy of thyroid myopathy. In: Gardner J, Vaughn V, Powell L (eds). Thyroid eye disease. Baltimore: Williams & Wilkins 1985; 207-18.

40. Hudson L, Feldon SE. Late overcorrection of hypotropia on Graves' ophthalmopathy. Ophthalmology 1992; 99:356-360.

41. Aust W, Schönherr F. Schieloperationen bei endokrin bedingten motilitätsstörungen. Ophthalmologica 1976; 173:171-179.

42. Boergen KP. Surgical repair of motility impairment in Graves' orbitopathy. Doc Ophthalmol 1989; 20:159-168.

43. Rüssmann W. Lähmungserscheinungen bei endokriner Orbitopathie-diagnostik und Therapie. Sitzungsber Ver Rhein-Westf Augenärzte 1980; 139:19-25.

44. Esser J. Graves' disease. Eye muscle surgery. Ophthalmologe 1994; 91:3-19.

45. Schimek RA. Surgical management of ocular complications of Graves' disease. Arch Ophthalmol 1972; 87:655-664.

46. Nardi M, Barca L. Hypercorrection of hypotropia in Graves' Ophthalmopathy. Ophthalmology 1993; 100:1-2.

47. Linberg JV, Anderson RL. Transorbital decompression. Arch Ophthalmol 1981; 99:113-119.
48. McCord CD. Orbital decompression for Graves' disease. Exposure through lateral canthal and inferior fornix incision. Ophthalmology 1981; 88:533-541.
49. McCord CD. Current trends in orbital decompression. Ophthalmology 1985; 92:21-33.
50. Hurwitz JJ, Birt D. An individualized approach to orbital decompression in Graves' orbitopathy. Arch Ophthalmol 1985; 103:660-665.
51. Leatherbarrow B, Lendrum J, Mahaffey PJ, Noble JL, Kwartz J, Davies H. Three wall orbital decompression for Graves' ophthalmopathy via a coronal approach. Eye 1991; 5:456-465.
52. Kao SCS, Chang T, Hou P. Surgical management of Graves 'ophthalmopathy. Stage I, inferomedial orbital decompression. J Formosan Med Ass 1992; 91:1154-1161.
53. Garrity JA, Fatourechi V, Bergstralh EJ, Bartley GB, Beatty ChW, Desanto LW, Gorman CA. Results of transantral orbital decompression in 428 patients with severe Graves' ophthalmopathy. Am J Ophthalmol 1993; 116:533-547.
54. Fatourechi V, Garrity JA, Bartley GB, Bergstralh EJ, DeSanto LW, Gorman CA. Graves ophthalmopathy. Results of transantral orbital decompression performed primarily for cosmetic indications. Ophthalmology 1994; 101:938-942.
55. Lyons ChJ, Rootman J. Orbital decompression for disfiguring exophthalmos in thyroid orbitopathy. Ophthalmology 1994; 101:223-230.
56. Kalmann R, Mourits MPh, van der Pol JP, Koornneef L. Coronal approach for rehabilitative orbital decompression in Graves' ophthalmopathy. Br J Ophthalmolol 1997; 81:41-45.
57. Paridaens DM, Van Buitenen HK, Mourits MPh. The incidence of diplopia following coronal and translid orbital decompression in Graves' orbitopathy. Eye 1998; 12:800-805.

4.   EYE LID SURGERY

Eyelid swelling and retraction are the most frequent abnormalities seen in GO,[1,2] and responsible for both functional (retraction, lagophthalmos) and cosmetic (swelling) complaints. In most healthy individuals, the upper lid covers the cornea at the 12 o'clock position for about 0.5 to 1.5 mm, whereas the lower lid margin touches the inferior corneal limbus.[3] In GO patients the upper lid is often found well above the upper part of the corneal limbus. Lid retraction enhances the proptotic appearance (pseudoproptosis) and together with infrequent blinking (Stellwag's sign) causes instability of the tear film covering the cornea, which in turn may lead to 'ocular discomfort', excessive lacrimation, photophobia, punctate keratitis or corneal ulceration. Upper lid retraction is seen especially at the lateral part of the upper lid.

As we have seen above lower lid retraction occurs as a complication of inferior rectus recession, but can also be part of the restrictive changes of the disease process itself. Eyelid swelling during the active stage of the disease can be caused by fluid accumulation. In the quiescent stage of the disease it is caused by an increase of preaponeutic and sometimes subdermal fat. This increase of tissue may alter the anatomical relationship of the two lamellae of which the eyelids consists, thereby causing ectropion or entropion. Not infrequently, the lid swelling is so severe, that the skin is pushed against the glasses, making the spectacle surface oily and reducing vision.

Lid retraction is treated with lid lengthening, of which many techniques have been described. Eyelid swelling is treated with blepharoplasty procedures, that do not differ from ordinary dermatochalasis corrections, with the exception that more fat is removed. Lid lengthening can be performed as an isolated procedure or combined with a blepharoplasty. For the sake of convenience, these will be discussed separately now. Tarsorrhaphy as a single procedure to reduce the lid aperture in GO is obsolete as the result is generally poor. However, a small tarsorrhaphy in combination with lid lengthening procedures can add the final touch to get an excellent result. Laser resurfacing of the skin, now an integral part of esthetic surgery, is a promising new tool in the cosmetic rehabilitation of the Graves' patient. Finally, botulinum toxin injections temporarily stretch glabellar furrows, which often disfigure the face in GO, and may also be used as a temporary chemodenervation of the upper lid retractors in the treatment of upper lid retraction.[4]

4.1   Upper lid retraction

4.1.1   Etiology

Upper lid retraction may vary from second to second depending upon the patient's state of consciousness and emotion. In many patients upper lid retraction disappears during the course of the ophthalmopathy, whereas in other patients with seemingly quiescent ophthalmopathy the amount of retraction increases. Eyelid swelling sometimes masks lid retraction, which then becomes visible after blepharoplasty. Lid retraction can also be masked by the GO patient's ability of pinching the eyes in order to compensate for the increased eye aperture and its consequences. A number of explanations for upper lid retraction in GO have been proposed:

1. Increased sympathetic tone as in thyrotoxicosis by which Müller's muscle is overstimulated, resulting in 1-2 mm rise of the upper lid. Increased sympathetic tone can, therefore, only be responsible for minor degrees of retraction. Guanethidine (postganglionic blocker) eyedrops have been used to counteract the increased sympathetic tone, but are of little value in most patients.

2. Contracture of the inferior rectus muscle increases the tone of the superior rectus muscle and of the levator palpebrae and, consequently, can cause upper lid retraction which will disappear after recession of the inferior rectus. "Fixation duress" refers to upper lid retraction while

fixing with an eye with inferior rectus muscle restriction due to excessive simultaneous firing of the ipsilateral superior rectus and levator palpebrae muscles. Fixation duress plays a significant role in upper lid retraction in GO in a subset of patients with restriction of the inferior rectus muscle.5

3. In patients operated because of long existing (>1 yr) upper lid retraction, fibrotic adhesions in the lacrimal gland area, around the levator itself, between the aponeurosis and the periosteum of the superior orbital margin, and fibrotic changes between conjunctiva and Müller's muscle are found and held responsible for the retraction.

4. Proptosis

4.1.2 Differential diagnosis

GO is the most frequent cause of upper lid retraction. However, it is also seen after trauma of the upper eyelid, after surgery of the upper eyelid (especially ptosis surgery), in neurologic diseases (e.g. Parinaud's syndrome), and constitutionally.

4.1.3 Indications for surgical correction of upper lid retraction

1) To reduce corneal exposure: sandy feeling, photophobia, tearing, keratitis, corneal ulcer; 2) for cosmetic rehabilitation; 3) to camouflage proptosis; 4) to prevent globe luxation. Because hyperthyroidism causes lid retraction, surgery should not be performed before the patient is euthyroid. Obviously the disease should have reached the quiescent stage with all symptoms and signs stable for at least 6 months. If orbital decompression and/or strabismus surgery is indicated, it should be done first.[6] Patients with corneal ulcers, however, should not follow these rules, but operated immediately to prevent corneal perforation.

4.1.4 Criteria to evaluate lid lengthening to correct upper retraction

Numerous techniques have been described to lengthen the upper lid in GO and Table 4 supplies an overview of contemporary techniques. For cosmetic reasons, a technique is required that sets and maintains the height and the contour of the eyelid within an accuracy of 1 mm, otherwise the result is an over- or undercorrection or an unacceptable lid contour. The effects of local anaesthetics, the use of adrenaline, perioperative haemorrhage, wound healing, Hering's law, and even of altered postoperative orbicularis and frontalis tone may annul the efforts.[7] In Table 4 criteria for evaluation of upper lid lengthening are suggested.

Table 4. Suggestions for the evaluation of upper eye lid lengthening

Result	Criteria
Perfect	1. The upper 0.5 -1.5 mm of the cornea in the 12 hrs position is covered by the eyelid.
	2. The difference in lid aperture between the left and right side is ≤ 1 mm.
	3. The patient is completely satisfied
	4. The lid margin contour is smooth
	5. The lid crease is within 7-10 mm of the lid margin.
	6. The skin fold of both lids is symmetrical
Acceptable	1. The upper eyelid margin is within 0.5 mm of the limbus, or covers no more than 2 mm of the cornea in the 12 o'clock position.
	2. The difference in lid aperture between the left and right is less than 2 mm.
	3. The patient is satisfied and demands no further treatment.
	4. As in perfect result 4-6
Failure	One or more of the above mentioned criteria are not fulfilled

4.1.5   Surgical technique for upper lid lengthening

We prefer local anesthesia and an operation table that can be placed electrically in upright position, this allowing us to ask the patient to open and close the eyes and to check the position of the upper lids in upright position, which may be markedly lower than in supine position. After infiltration with approximately 2 cc of prilocaine 1% together with epinephrine 1/200,000 subcutaneously, a lid crease incision is made through skin and orbicularis muscle. The orbital septum is opened and the levator aponeurosis and muscle identified. Adhesions are cut and excessive preaponeurotic fat excised using bipolar or monopolar cautery.

The lateral horn is cut completely along the medial side of the lacrimal gland. The levator aponeurosis together with Müller's muscle is stripped from the conjunctiva and the lateral part of the tarsal plate as far medially until an acceptable position of the eyelid (the patient in upright position) has been reached. Using epinephrine, the ideal position is when the upper lid touches the upper corneal limbus, as a further drop of 0.5-1.5 mm can be expected when the epinephrine has worn off. To prevent further spontaneous disinsertion, a 6.0 nylon suture is placed through the upper horizontal middle of the tarsal plate and sutured on a loop to the detached aponeurosis.

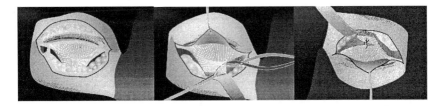

Figure 12. Technique for upper lid lengthening, seen from the surgeons' perspective. (Contributed by M.Ph. Mourits)[7]

Table 5. Results of upper lid lenghtening procedures in Graves' ophthalmopathy (satisf, satisfactory; acc, acceptable). Other publications which are not included.[8-11,15,16]

Author	Type of surgery	Nr of patients/lids	Results
Putterman[12]	Graded Müllerotomy +/- levator aponeurosis recession	32/53	Success: 81%
Doxanas[13]	Sclera interposition	/18	Success: 61%
Harvey[14]	Müllerectomy, levator recession, lateral horn cut	14/24	Good-acc: 76% Failures: 24%
Thaller[17]	Müller recession	11/	Acc: 73%
	Levator recession	30/	Acc: 89%
	Levator recession + sclera	13/	Acc: 89%
	Z-myotomy	5/	Acc 100%
Hedin[18]	Müllerectomy + levator division	27/40	Acc: 90%
Harvey[19]	Recession levator, Müller	12/22	Good: 86%
Levine[20]	Recession levator, Müller	15/	Success: 87%
Mourits[3]	Sclera interposition	47/78	Acc: 77%
Liu[21]	Central aponeurosis disinsertion	9/	Satisf: 77%
Uccello[22]	Free levator complex recession	11/	Acc: 73%
Ceisler[23]	Müllerotomy + levator aponeurosis transposition	37/72	Acc: 98%
Tucker[24]	Adjustable levator recession	/9	Good: 60-75%
	Nonadjustable levator recession	/73	Good: 32-34%
Woog[25]	Adjustable levator recession	9/12	Acc: 86%
Mourits[7]	Lateral levator recession, Müller	50/78	Acc: 82%

Using this technique in 78 upper lids of 50 consecutive patients with upper lid retraction varying from 1 to 7 mm from the corneal limbus, a perfect and stable result (see criteria) was achieved in 50% and an acceptable in another 32% of the patients. Most surgeons agree that detachment of the lateral horn of the aponeurosis is crucial in upper lid lengthening. Some surgeons use different techniques for different degrees of lid retraction (Müllerectomy for minor degrees of retraction; a combined Müllerectomy plus levator aponeurosis recession in more advanced forms of lid retraction) and some prefer adjustable sutures or use small modifications (Table 5). The use of sclera, popular in the Eighties, has been abandoned, because scleral interposition does not increase the success rate.

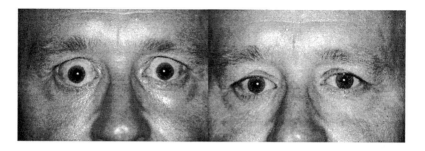

Figure 13. A patient before and after upper lid lengthening using the above described technique. Reproduced with permission from the patient. (Contributed by M.Ph. Mourits)

4.1.6   Complications

Common are undercorrection (especially at the lateral side), overcorrection (which usually troubles the patient more than undercorrection), asymmetry, and a high lid crease. We have never seen the possible complication of transection of lacrimal ductules with a resulting dry eye. However, we found iatrogenic ptosis after eyelid lengthening more difficult to correct than blepharoptosis originating from other causes.

4.2   Lower lid retraction

4.2.1   Etiology

1. Increased sympathetic tone (thyrotoxicosis); 2. Contracture of the superior rectus muscle; 3. Inferior rectus recession; 4. Fibrosis; 5. Proptosis. To prevent lower lid retraction after inferior rectus muscle recession, dissection of fascial connections around the inferior rectus muscle is advocated.[26] Meyer *et al.*[27] described a technique of 'infratarsal lower eyelid retractor lysis' to overcome lower lid retraction.

4.2.2   Indications for surgery, evaluation of results

The indications for lower lid retraction are similar as for upper lid retraction. A perfect result is a lower lid with a smooth contour, touching the corneal limbus at the 6 o'clock position.

4.2.3 Surgical technique and results

Whereas the use of spacers in upper lid retraction does not increase the predictability of the outcome, it is commonly agreed that spacers are required for more severe forms of lower lid lengthening. This is due to the effect of gravity in upright position, reducing the efficacy of lower lid surgery. After infiltration with prilocaine 1% with epinephrine 1/200,000 subconjunctivally, the conjunctiva is incised over the lower border of the tarsal plate. The lower lid retractors are identified and dissected off the conjunctiva and the tarsus and freed of the orbital septum. A spacer of about three times the amount of lid retraction in millimeters is sutured to the retractors and the tarsus. The conjunctiva is left as it is or closed with a running Vicryl suture.

Spacers used for lower lid lengthening are: donor sclera, Vicryl mesh, cartilage, and hard palate mucosa. Sclera has some tendency to retract. Conchal cartilage is a good spacer, but should be thinned very carefully, because otherwise it is too stifff. Cohen *et al.*[28] described good and lasting results in three out of four eyelids lengthened with hard palate mucosa grafts. In contrast, Feldman *et al.*[29] modified their original technique consisting of scleral implant lengthening with a lateral tarsal strip and/or lateral tarsorrhaphy, because of persistent retraction. Using sclera only, our success rate (good + acceptable results) after one operation was almost 90%.[3]

4.2.4 Complications

Coomon is undercorrection, or recurrence of retraction. Complications of inserting a spacer are: extrusion, shrinkage or migration of the spacer, thick eyelid, cyst formation, wound infection and granuloma.

4.3 Blepharoplasty and fat removal

Blepharoplasty is the final surgical procedure in the functional and cosmetic rehabilitation of the GO-patient. The lid crease is marked and the amount of redundant skin estimated having the patient in upright position. After infiltration with local anesthetics, the redundant skin is excised using a knife, a laser, or monopolar cauterization needle. In the upper eyelid, the skin excision may be generous, although not excessive. In the lower lid, the skin excision should be modest to avoid lower lid retraction or ectropion. To get satisfying results, it is important to remove the preaponeurotic fat extensively and even subdermal fat together with orbicularis fibers. Bulging fat of the lower lids can also be removed through a transconjunctival incision in patients without excess of skin.

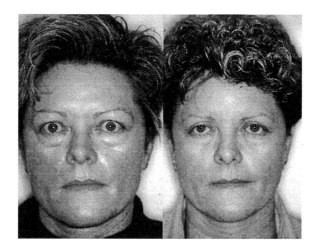

Figure 14. An ophthalmopathy patient before (left) and after (right) upper plus lower lid blepharoplasty plus an upper lid lengthening. Reproduced with permission from the patient. (Contributed by M.Ph. Mourits)

4.4   Adjuvant procedures

New developments in aesthetic surgery find their way into oculoplastic rehabilitative surgery. These include the use of a CO_2-laser for skin resurfacing and flattening of skinfolds and crow's feet and lifting of the Sub-Orbicularis Oculi Fat (SOOF).

4.5   References

1. Day RM. Ocular manifestations of thyroid disease: current concepts. Tr Am Ophthalmol Soc 1959; 57:572-601.
2. Bartley GB. The epidemiologic characteristics and clinical course of ophthalmopathy associated with autoimmune thyroid disease in Olmsted county, Minnesota. Trans Am Ass Ophthalmol 1994; 92:477-588.
3. Mourits MP, Koornneef L. Lid lengthening by sclera interposition for eyelid retraction in Graves' ophthalmopathy. Br J Ophthalmol 1991; 75:344-347.
4. Özkam SB, Can D, Söylev MF, Arsan AK, Duman S. Chemodenervation in the treatment of upper eyelid retraction. Ophthalmologica 1997; 211:387-390.
5. Hamed LF, Lessner AM. Fixation duress in the pathogenesis of upper eyelid retraction in thyroid orbitopathy. Ophthalmology 1994; 101:1608-1613.
6. Frueh BR, Musch DC, Garber FW. Lid retraction and levator aponeurosis defects in Graves' eye disease. Ophthalmic Surg 1986; 17:216-220.
7. Mourits MP, Sasim IV. A single technique to correct various degrees of upper lid retraction in patients with Graves' orbitopathy. Br J Ophthalmol 1999; 83:81-84.
8. Henderson JW. Relief of eyelid retraction. Arch Ophthalmol 1965; 74:205-216.
9. Putterman AM, Urist M. Surgical treatment of upper eyelid retraction. Arch Ophthalmol 1972; 87:401-405.

10. Baylis HI, Cies WA, Kamin DF. Correction of upper lid retraction,. Am J Ophthalmol 1976; 82:790-794.
11. Dryden RM, Soll DB. The use of scleral transplantation in cicatricial entropion and eyelid retraction. Tr Am Acad Ophth & Otol 1977; 83: 669-678.
12. Putterman AM. Graded Müller's muscle excision and levator recession. Am J Ophthalmol 1981; 88:507-512.
13 Doxanas MT, Dryden RM. The use of sclera in the treatment of dysthyroid eyelid retraction. Ophthalmology 1981; 88:887-894.
14. Harvey JT, Anderson RL. The aponeurotic approach to eyelid retraction. Ophthalmology 1981; 88:513-524.
15. Grove AS. Upper eyelid retraction and Graves' disease. Am J Ophthalmol 1981; 88:499-507.
16. Grove AS. Upper eyelid retraction: Treatment by levator marginal myotomy. Orbit 1982; 1:21-31.
17. Thaller VT, Kaden K, Lane CM, Collin JRO. Thyroid lid surgery. Eye 1987; 1:609-614.
18. Hedin A. Eyelid surgery in dysthyroid ophthalmopathy. Eye 1988; 2:201-206.
19. Harvey JT, Corin S, Nixon D, Veloudios A. Modified levator aponeurosis recession for upper eyelid retraction in Graves' disease. Ophthalmic Surg 1991; 22:313-217.
20. Levine MR, Chu A. Surgical treatment of thyroid-related lid retraction: a new variation. Ophthalmic Surg 1991; 22:90-94.
21. Liu D. Surgical correction of upper lid retraction. Ophthalmic Surg 1993; 24:323-327.
22. Ucello G, Vassallo P, Strianes D, Bonavolontà G. Free levator complex recession in Graves' ophthalmopathy. Orbit 1994; 13:119-122.
23 Ceisler EJ, Bilyk JR, Rubin PAD, Burks WR, Shore JW. Results of Müllerotomy and levator aponeurosis transposition for the correction of upper lid retraction in Graves' disease. Ophthalmology 1995; 102:483-492.
24. Tucker SM, Collin R. Repair of upper eyelid retraction: a comparison between adjustable and non-adjustable sutures. Br J Ophthalmol 1995; 79:658-660.
25. Woog JL, Hartstein ME, Hoenig J. Adjustable suture technique for levator recession. Arch Ophthalmol 1996; 114:620-624.
26. Kushner BJ. A surgical procedure to minimize lower eyelid retraction with inferior rectus recession. Arch Ophthalmol 1992; 101:1011-1014.
27. Meyer DR, Simon JW, Kansora M. Primary infratarsal lower eyelid retractor lysis to prevent eyelid retraction after inferior rectus muscle recession. Am J Ophthalmol 1996; 122:331-339.
28 Cohen MS, Shorr N. Eyelid reconstruction with hard palate mucosa grafts. Ophalmic Plast Reconstr Surg 1992; 8:183-195.
29. Feldman KA, Putterman AMM, Farber MD. Surgical treatment of thyroid-related lower eyelid retraction: a modified approach. Ophthalmic Plast Reconstr Surg 1992; 8:278-286.

Chapter 10

Future Research in Graves' ophthalmopathy

Hemmo A. Drexhage,* Anthony P. Weetman, Armin E. Heufelder, Steve E. Feldon, Leo Koornneef, Maarten Ph. Mourits, Wilmar M. Wiersinga, Mark F. Prummel.

Department of Immunology, Erasmus University Rotterdam, PO Box 1738, 3000 DR Rotterdam, The Netherlands

Graves' eye disease is characterized by a chronic round cell infiltrate of the retrobulbar tissues (sometimes of focal character and organized in T cell zones and B cell follicles[1]) and a very strong association with Graves' thyroid disease. The latter is an accepted autoimmune disease and caused by autoantibodies (Abs) against the TSH-receptor (TSH-R), which stimulate thyrocytes to grow and to produce excessive amounts of thyroid hormones. On the basis of its histology and the association with Graves' thyroid disease it has for long been the idea that Graves' eye disease is of autoimmune character too, and that the TSH-R is an important antigen also in the pathogenesis of the eye signs. This chapter tries to summarize recent developments in endocrine autoimmunity in general and Graves' ophthalmopathy in particular.

1. FUTURE RESEARCH ON THE EXPRESSION OF THE TSH-R IN THE ORBIT

Despite intensive research, the identity and nature of the principle target autoantigen in Graves' eye disease is still unclear. One or two decades ago it was thought that the primary autoimmune reaction was directed against antigens specific for eye muscle cells. Indeed autoantibodies against muscle cells in general and autoantibodies against a 64 kD eye muscle protein were detected in the serum of Graves' ophthalmopathy patients.[2,3] Recently this latter autoantigen turned out to be the flavoprotein subunit of mitochondrial succinate dehydrogenase.[4]

Presently the idea is favored that the eye muscle damage and the eye muscle autoimmune reaction are secondary to a primary autoimmune reaction directed to orbital connective tissue and fat cells. Also for this view evidence was given some decades ago in experiments showing that the TSH-R was not only functionally expressed on thyrocytes, but also on some special fat cells.[5] Moreover TSH-R antibody preparations derived from the serum of patients with Graves' ophthalmopathy were able to stimulate collagen synthesis in cultured fibroblasts.[6] These early data remained conjectural, since many hesitated (due to the technical flaws of the experiments of those days) to accept the idea that the TSH-R was functionally expressed on cells other than thyrocytes. Moreover not every research group was able to repeat the fibroblast stimulating experiments using purified Graves' immunoglobulin preparations. However, due to improved molecular techniques to express the TSH-R in culture cell systems, to reliably measure its mRNA expression, and to raise monoclonal antibodies (BA8, 3G4) for detection in conventional immunohistochemistry, new approaches have used to tackle the old questions. The idea is presently gaining momentum that an autoimmune reaction to an extrathyroidally expressed TSH-R forms the cornerstone in the pathogenesis of Graves' eye disease. Using Northern blotting and immunohistochemistry, the TSH-R has been found on 'preadipocytic fibroblasts' and on adipocytes in the retrobulbar fat and the perimysium of extra-ocular muscles particularly of Graves' ophthalmopathy patients.[7,8] The functionality of the TSH-R on such "preadipocytic fibroblasts" was shown in experiments where TSH induced c-AMP signals in "differentiated orbital preadipocytes".[9] The questions remaining for future research in this area are:

> Which fibroblastic cells exactly express the TSH-R, or, in other words, what are the characteristics of 'preadipocytic orbital fibroblasts'? Is it possible that all fibroblasts under certain circumstances start to express the TSH-R, or are there only specific subtypes of fibroblasts capable of expressing the TSH-R? Are these cells expressing TSH-R located in the extra-ocular muscles?

> Is the TSH-R expressed on "preadipocytic fibroblasts" in the same form as on thyrocytes, or as isoforms or parts of the TSH-R?

> What are the effects of TSH stimulation or thyroid stimulating antibodies on such 'TSH-R positive preadipocytic fibroblasts' not only in terms of further differentiation into adipocytes, but also in terms of the synthesis of important mediators of edema formation?

2. FUTURE RESEARCH ON ANIMAL MODELS OF GRAVES' DISEASE AND GRAVES' EYE DISEASE

If Graves' ophthalmopathy is to be considered an autoimmune disease, it does not suffice to only detect a putative autoantigen. Koch's postulates also demand that:

– An immune reaction towards such autoantigen should be detected (in intensity correlating to the severity of the disease),
– Via immunization with the autoantigen, the disease can be elicited in a non-affected host, and/or that transfer of the (elicited) specific autoreactive immune components - be it immune serum or immune cells - precipitates a disease in the recipient.

Regarding the requirement for the presence of an autoimmune reaction towards the TSH-R, it is common knowledge that many of the Graves' ophthalmopathy patients have antibodies to the receptor, often in high titers. There are also recent reports using the purified extracellular domain of the human TSH-R expressed as a fusion protein (MBP-ECD) and Western blotting techniques that show that those ophthalmopathy patients who do not have TSH-R Abs by conventional methods, show TSH-R reactive IgG and IgA antibodies,[10] although, admittedly, also some healthy controls are positive when using these approaches. Future research must therefore aim at devising techniques to obtain sufficient human TSH-R protein to develop assays to quantitatively measure TSH-R antibodies and their subclasses.

With regard to the other requirement of Koch's postulate, considerable progress has been made over the last couple of years. Actually Koch's postulates have been fulfilled almost completely. It has been proven possible to elicit in female BALB/C mice a mild Graves' like disease using vaccinations with MBP-ECD.[11] A slightly raised serum thyroxin level characterized the immunized mice and they became TBII positive. Upon transfer of splenic lymphocytes of these 'experimental allergic Graves' disease' mice to naive female BALB/C mice, the recipients developed mild orbital changes suggestive of Graves' ophthalmopathy, with an endomysial edema and a round cell and mast cell infiltration of the eye muscles.[11] Of note in these transfer experiments is firstly that it was not the TSH-R autoantibodies but rather the lymphocytes which were the mediators of the eye disease, and secondly that the Graves' like phenomena were strain-specific (i.e. genetically restricted) in that the vaccination and transfer protocol carried out in NOD mice did not result in hyperthyroidism and eye signs, but in destructive thyroiditis only. Since BALB/C mice are TH2-skewed animals while NOD mice are TH1-skewed, the data suggest that TSH-R specific TH2 cells are involved in orbital pathology. Moreover, the infiltration pattern in the BALB/C thyroiditis indeed suggested a TH2 reaction, with B cells being more numerous than T cells, and a cytokine profile of high IL-4/IFNγ ratios.

The testable hypothesis thus is that TSH-R's (or peptides thereof) derived from fibroblasts, preadipocytes and/or adipocytes interact with sensitized TH2 cells in the retrobulbar space. The sequelae of such interaction should then lead to signs and symptoms of the eye disease. Using this transfer model, it is now possible to investigate the effector mechanisms of the immune reaction in the retrobulbar space. The main questions are:

Are TH2 cells indeed involved, and what are the specific TH2 cytokines/chemokines or adhesive interactions of TH2 cells with TSH-R expressing 'preadipocytic fibroblasts'/adipocytes resulting in an altered growth rate and metabolism of these target cells?

What is the additional role - if any - of TSH-R Abs in this TH2 mediated interaction (blocking or aggravation of the disease, and do they elicit the TSH-R on "preadipocytic fibroblasts")?

The drawback of the presently developed BALB/C transfer model is that the orbital pathology is very mild. There is thus room for improvements. Other approaches that give more vigorous immune responses should be carried out. In this respect, data are awaited from yet another mouse model of Graves' disease, namely immunization of AKR/N mice with MHC-class II and TSH-R expressing fibroblasts.[12] In this latter model it was shown that particularly the N terminal part of the TSH-R was of importance in eliciting a Graves'-like disease.[13] Further developments of TSH-R gene vaccination,[14] and TSH-R vaccinations enforced by professional APCs, such as the dendritic cells[15] are indicated.

3.   FUTURE RESEARCH ON TARGET AND IMMUNE ABNORMALITIES

Recent research in the field of type 1 diabetes aims at the prediction and prevention of the disease. For the purpose of prediction, large-scale studies have been started in healthy first-degree relatives of probands with type 1 diabetes.[16] In these relatives (with a high risk of developing the disease), the value of different varieties of islet reactive autoantibodies to predict the outbreak of disease has been determined. To enable further improvements in this prediction, and to devise prevention strategies, it is important to be informed on the immune cellular aspects of the early, non-clinical stages of the disease. The study of animal models of spontaneously developing forms of endocrine autoimmune disease has proven to be of value in this respect.

The BB rat spontaneously develops autoimmune insulitis/diabetes, and a small goiter with intrathyroidal lymphoid tissue. The NOD mouse spontaneously develops autoimmune insulitis/diabetes and a Sjögren-like syndrome, but hardly thyroid autoimmune disease (except for some strains). The OS chicken spontaneously develops Hashimoto-like hypothyroidism.

The evidence obtained in all three animal models points in one direction: the endocrine autoimmune diseases are multifactorial and multigenic in origin. There is thus no simple cause for the diseases, and only unfortunate combinations of various disease-promoting and disease-protecting genes together with eliciting endogenous and environmental factors lead to clinically overt disease. It is thus no surprise that the development of endocrine autoimmune diseases is complex and often a prolonged process.

Various disease stages can be discerned. Fig. 1 shows an example of such staging based on the classical division of immune responses in an afferent, central and efferent immune response. In the afferent immune response, antigen is transported from the periphery to the draining lymph nodes to be presented to the locally accumulated, naive lymphocytes. In the central immune reaction, a specific immune response is elicited in the naive lymphocytes resulting in the generation of antibodies and specific effector T cells. The efferent immune reaction or effector response is due to the effects of the specific antibodies and specific effector T cells on their target. In essence, thyroid autosensitization in the BB rat and the NOD mouse follows the same pattern (Fig. 2). The animal models of spontaneously developing endocrine autoimmune disease have shown that in each of these stages of the 'autoreactive immune response', various, non-mutually exclusive aberrations from normal can be detected, which apparently in combination lead to an excessive and inappropriate immune reaction towards self (Fig. 3). In essence and in summary: multiple target abnormalities together with multiple immunodysregulations lead to wrong setpoints in immune cell-target interaction with pathology as consequence.

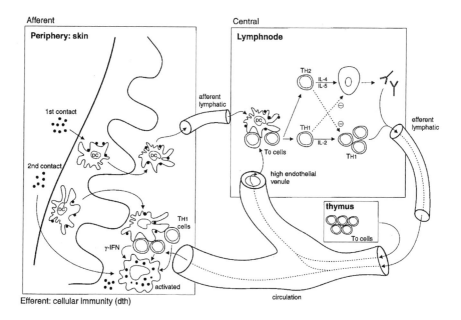

Figure 1 A schematic (simplified) view of a normal immune response elicited via the skin and resulting in a delayed type hypersensitivity (DTH) reaction, e.g. a tuberculin reaction. The response is divided in an afferent, central and efferent phase.

Afferent phase: takes hours. Upon a first contact with the antigen PPD (•) specialized antigen presenting cells, such as the dendritic cells (DC) take up and process the antigen. DC travel with these PPD antigens via afferent lymph vessels to the draining lymph nodes, where they meet (amongst other cells) naïve (To) recirculating CD4+ T cells (originating in the thymus).

Central phase: takes 4-6 days. DC stimulate naive CD4$^+$ T cells with a receptor for PPD antigen to clonally expand, and direct (amongst other cells) the pathway of development of the clonally expanded PPD-specific T cells: either TH2 cells producing interleukin (IL)-4 and IL-5 for B cell help, or in this case of PPD sensitization TH1 cells capable of producing pro-inflammatory cytokines like γ-interferon (γ-IFN). IL-4 and IL-5 are instrumental in the maturation of plasma cells from B cells, which produce antibodies (YY). Both antigen-specific T cells and antibodies leave the lymph node 6-10 days after antigen challenge (via the efferent lymphatic or the blood stream) to circulate in the now immunized host.

Efferent phase: upon a second contact with the antigen (or when the antigen persists) sensitized TH1 cells are able to interact locally in the skin with PPD antigen-bearing DC. Upon production of γ-IFN, macrophages are activated and also other factors are produced causing a specific local inflammatory reaction, i.e. the delayed tuberculin reaction (erythema, edema and round cell infiltration at 48-96 hrs after 2nd antigen challenge).

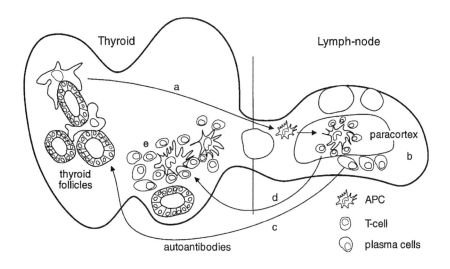

Figure 2. A schematic representation of a thyroid autoimmune reaction divided in an afferent, central and efferent phase like a normal immune reaction. See for parallels Fig.1.

Afferent phase: DC start to accumulate in the thyroid and autoantigenic peptides (from Tg, TPO and perhaps the TSH-R) are later transported with the DC to the draining lymph nodes.

Central phase: various thyroid autoantigen-specific T cells are clonally expanded and B cells differentiate into plasma cells producing thyroid reactive autoantibodies;

Efferent phase I: thyroid reactive autoantibodies have their effect on the thyrocytes (destruction, stimulation/blockade of growth and function); Efferent phase II: thyroid reactive T cells have their local effects, e.g., a DTH-like, TH1 effect (destruction of thyrocytes via activated macrophages) or, efferent phase III: the development of a local lymphoid tissue.

4. FUTURE RESEARCH ON ABNORMALITIES IN THE AFFERENT PHASE OF THE IMMUNE REACTION

The histomorphological hallmark of the abnormal afferent immune reaction in all three animal models of spontaneously developing endocrine autoimmunity is an enhanced accumulation of antigen-presenting dendritic cells (DC) and macrophages (MØ) in the target-tissue-to-be.[17] There are various conditions that may lead to this accumulation. Firstly, classical inflammatory triggers accompanying an early non-specific necrosis of thyrocytes or β cells (by iodine intoxication or streptozotocin) induce a non-specific leucocytic infiltration, initially of polymorphonuclear leukocytes, later replaced by lymphocytes, macrophages and dendritic cells.[18]

There is, however, also another putative mechanism for DC and MØ accumulation in the target-organ-to-be. To understand this mechanism, it is important to realize that DCs and MØ are in fact a normal component of endocrine glands. The cells are present in relatively low numbers in normal thyroids and in normal islets, but in relatively high numbers in the normal anterior pituitary (called folliculo-stellate cells) and in the ovary and testis.[19] Upon isolation such DC are able to down regulate the growth and hormone production of neighboring endocrine cells in vitro.[20,21] They exert such endocrine regulatory functions via brief clustering interactions with the endocrine cells while delivering cytokine signals such as IL-1β and IL-6. Also in vivo there is an indication of such endocrine regulatory role of monocyte derived cells in the islets of Langerhans; prevention of monocyte infiltration into islets by depletion experiments in a transgenic mouse model of diabetes resulted in a slight, but consistent rise in the proliferation of ductal and islet cells.[22] It is thus possible that the very early accumulation of DC in endocrine tissues, that are the later targets of an autoimmune response, could be the consequence of early metabolic or growth alterations of the endocrine cells, making a regulatory influx of DC necessary. Indeed, numerous reports show that OS chicken thyroids,[23] BB rat thyroids,[24] BB rat islets,[25] NOD mouse islets[26] and NOD mouse salivary glands[27] are inherently abnormal in their growth as well as in their hormone or oxidative radical production at the time of early DC accumulation. Such metabolic and growth abnormalities are also present in the islets and salivary glands of the SCID-variants of the animal models[26,27] showing that T and B lymphocytes can be ruled out as initiators of such early pre-autoimmune glandular abnormalities. It is likely that such early growth and metabolic abnormalities of the pre-autoimmune endocrine glands not only attract DC but also have repercussions on the de novo expression of relevant autoantigens,[28] e.g. important enzymes and receptors.

This phenomenon of early DC infiltration for the purpose of endocrine regulation (Fig. 3) also explains the mild, non-destructive thyroid autoimmune sensitization occurring in iodine-deficient humans and rats.[29-31] When iodine deficient goiter develops, DC start to infiltrate the goitrous gland in both humans and rats,[31,32] presumably to regulate the enhanced growth rate and oxidative radical production of the iodine-deficient thyrocytes. In the rats the DC infiltration is followed in time by a relatively mild production of anti-colloid antibodies and a relatively mild infiltration with single, isolated lymphocytes.[31] Apparently concomitant abnormalities in immunoregulation are required for an excessive, pathologic anti-colloid antibody production and a development of an abnormal lymphocytic thyroiditis to follow such an initial DC infiltration (Fig. 3). Indeed mild iodine deficiency in the autoimmune-prone BB-DP rat leads to an acceleration and aggravation of the autoimmune thyroiditis process as compared to the process in the iodine sufficient BB rat (unpublished data).

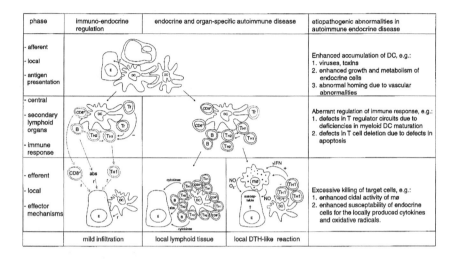

phase	immuno-endocrine regulation	endocrine and organ-specific autoimmune disease	etiopathogenic abnormalities in autoimmune endocrine disease
- afferent - local - antigen presentation			Enhanced accumulation of DC, e.g.: 1. viruses, toxins 2. enhanced growth and metabolism of endocrine cells 3. abnormal homing due to vascular abnormalities
- central - secondary lymphoid organs - immune response			Aberrant regulation of immune response, e.g.: 1. defects in T regulator circuits due to deficiencies in myeloid DC maturation 2. defects in T cell deletion due to defects in apoptosis
- efferent - local - effector mechanisms			Excessive killing of target cells, e.g.: 1. enhanced cidal activity of mø 2. enhanced susceptability of endocrine cells for the locally produced cytokines and oxidative radicals.
	mild infiltration	local lymphoid tissue	local DTH-like reaction

Figure 3. A similar schematic representation of a thyroid autoimmune reaction as in Fig. 2, but from a different perspective. More emphasis is put on the view that a 'physiologic' controlled thyroid autoimmunity may exist ('immuno-endocrine regulation in iodine deficiency), and that various aberrations from such a process of controlled immune reactivity may lead to pathology (see further text). E = endocrine cell, DC = dendritic cell, r = regulation, Tr = T regulator cells, abs = antibodies, Mφ = macrophage. See legend Figs. 1 and 2 for abbreviations.

5. FUTURE RESEARCH ON ABNORMALITIES IN THE CENTRAL PHASE OF THE IMMUNE REACTION

The hallmark of the abnormal central immune reaction in organ-specific endocrine autoimmunity is an inappropriate and excessive production of autoreactive effector T cells (both of TH1 and/or TH2 phenotype) and of autoantibodies. This inappropriate production is due to imbalances in the normally meticulously set, regulating network of various cross-talking cells of the immune system (Fig. 3).

In the BB-DP rat the immunoregulatory defects are linked to a severe lymphopenia which gradually develops in the animal from birth onwards. This lymphopenia is under control of the lyp-gene,[33] and predominantly affects the RT6+ T cell population. It is precisely this population of T cells that suppresses autoimmune responsiveness in the normal rat. Transfer at young age of RT6+ T cells from a nondiabetic rat to the BB-DP rat prevents the development of autoimmune insulitis and thyroiditis.[34] With regard to the origin of the lack of T cells, and predominantly of the regulatory RT6+ T cells, there are reports that BB-DP bone-marrow derived cells, that are not T cell precursors, influence the maturation environment in the thymus in such a way that faulty T cell development results.[35] These observations suggest an abnormal function of intrathymic DC and/or MØ, leading to abnormal T cell development.[36] With regard to DC at other sites in the BB rat than the thymus, we recently showed that splenic and lymph node DC of BB-DP rats have an immature phenotype from birth onwards and are very poor stimulators of the syngeneic (syn)-MLR[37] (syn-MLRs represent proliferative responses to self peptides). Particularly relevant are our observations that the immature DC were predominantly faulty in the generation of regulatory RT6+ T cells in such syn-MLR.[37] Interestingly, similar defects in DC maturation and function have been found in recent onset type 1 diabetic patients,[38] in recent onset autoimmune thyroiditis patients (to be published), and even in prediabetic individuals positive for islet cell antibodies.[39] Also the NOD mouse model is characterized by maturation defects in the lineage's of DC and MØ from bone marrow precursors (besides T cell apoptosis defects).[40]

It is thus not too daring a concept that disturbances in the maturation of myeloid DC and MØ exist in the BB-DP rat, the human, and the NOD mouse. The resulting abnormalities in DC and Mφ function probably lead to abnormalities in the conductance of the T cell orchestra by these cells, both at the level of the thymus and in the peripheral lymphoid tissues. These abnormalities in the conductance of the T cell orchestra result in its off-key tuning: an abundance of autoreactive effector T cells over that of regulator T cells.

The defective cross-talk between APCs and T cells is probably at least partly genetically determined, since there are strong associations between the occurrence of autoimmune insulitis and autoimmune thyroiditis and certain genes involved in such cross-talk, e.g. certain MHC-haplotypes (DR3-DQβ1*0201; DR3-DQα1*0501)[41,42] and costimulatory molecules (a microsatellite polymorphism of the CTLA-4 gene-alleles 106).[43,44] Besides these immune genes environmental factors must be involved in the hampered cross talk. Iodine, PCBs and viruses have all been reported as influencing DC and MØ development.[17] Obviously experiments need to be carried out to further detail the various DC, T cell and MØ abnormalities preceding and probably underlying organ-specific autoimmune reactions.

It remains to be seen whether Graves' thyroid disease and Graves' eye disease develop following the above described pattern. Here obviously the lack of a spontaneous animal model for Graves' disease pays its toll. In fact the site of afferent immune reactivity is fully unknown in Graves' disease. There are three possibilities:

The thyroid.

The fact that radio-iodine treatment of sporadic non-toxic goiter (a condition with raised numbers of intrathyroidal DC[45]) leads in some cases[46,47] to TSH-R Ab-positive hyperthyroidism (Graves' disease by definition) suggests that an increased thyrocyte decay and intrathyroidal autoantigen release (perhaps the TSH-R) in an appropriate microenvironment (raised numbers of DC) may be one of the driving forces behind the induction of an excessive immune reactivity towards the TSH-R (particularly in immune dysregulated individuals, see Fig.3). The aggravation of Graves' eye signs after radioiodine treatment of a Graves' goiter may be explained similarly.

The orbit.

Venous obstruction in the feline orbit has proven to precipitate a pathology that is similar to Graves' ophthalmopathy.[48] This "cat model" of Graves' eye disease, developed by Feldon, shows that venous stasis is an important factor for eliciting a retrobulbar inflammation due to local anoxia and hypercapnia. It may come as no surprise considering the above description that such a non-specific inflammation (also involving MHC class II[+] DC and MØ) could form the triggerpoint for an autosensitization towards preadipocytic fibroblasts particularly in organisms that are immune dysregulated (cats are often affected by feline leukemia virus, inducing a long preleukemic state of immune-dysregulation).[49] The cat model of Feldon clearly needs further investigation (Fig. 4), and opens possibilities to construct new animal models for Graves' eye disease, where local inflammatory abnormalities may bring out systemic immune dysregulation.

The gut

Yersinia *enterocolitica* shares epitopes with the TSH-R.[50,51] Will it also be possible to induce a mild Graves' like disease in female BALB/C mice via vaccinations with Y. *enterocolitica* instead of with TSH-R preparations? It must be noted in this respect that the gut microflora also plays an important role in the development of experimental allergic thyroiditis in the rat.[52] Perhaps just leakage of foreign antigens from the gut leads to other setpoints in the immune system?

With regard to the central autoimmune reaction, it is of note that Graves' patients show the same abnormalities in the function of their DC (maturation defects) and MΦ (enhanced oxygen radical, cytokine and prostaglandin production) as type 1 diabetics or autoimmune hypothyroid patients.[53] There are recent reports that serum levels of DC/Mφ cytokines such as IL-1 and IL-1RA[54,55] are also abnormal in Graves' disease. Future research must detail and expand these findings, and investigate whether serum cytokine determinations are helpful in clarifying the immune disturbance. If possible, results should be compared with orbital cytokine profiles.

Also efforts should be devoted to the genetic abnormalities in Graves' disease. Large scale (multicenter) studies are indicated to obtain sufficiently high numbers of sib pairs to trace the various genomic stretches related to the disease.[56] Alternatively, such studies could be carried out in closed communities. Of note is that there are genetic differences between the various forms of endocrine autoimmunity. Type 1 diabetes is clearly linked to DR3 and DR4 genes and in particular to DR4-DQB1*0302. Graves' disease shows only a modest linkage to DR3 genes with a low relative risk. This observation leaves sufficient space for increased research into the identification of environmental factors.

In the early nineties it was shown that T cell clones derived from Graves' orbital tissues were mainly CD8$^+$ T cells, and produced considerable amounts of IFN-γ next to IL-4 and IL-10.[57] These CD8$^+$ T cell clones reacted to autologous (but not allogeneic) retrobulbar fibroblasts with cell proliferation, but did not induce fibroblast destruction. It must be noted, however, that recent reports showed the opposite, namely a predominance of CD4$^+$ T cell clones.[58,59] These clones were not able to react to a retroocular muscle preparation, yet one reacted to a thyroid antigen preparation.[59] The clones produced a wide array of both TH1 and TH2 type cytokines. With regard to TCR-V gene usage retrobulbar T cell clones from recent onset eye disease show a restricted heterogeneity and share TCR-V gene usage with thyroid and pretibial T cell clones, giving a strong indication for shared antigens at these sites.[60]

With regards to the detection of endocrine autoantigen-specific T cells in the circulation, numerous studies have been carried out over the last 10-15 years, especially in recent onset type 1 diabetics, but also in Graves' eye disease. Using the conventional T cell proliferation assays driven by the various relevant autoantigens, it has become clear that healthy individuals also harbor such autoantigen specific T cells, and that the frequency of such autoreactive T cells is only marginally raised in patients. It is presently assumed that the presence of autoreactive T cells is not abnormal in itself, but that the skewing of these T cells has shifted patients from protective (TH3, perhaps TH2) to aggressive (TH1) immunity. Whether this is reflected by an altered T cell cytokine balance in autoantigen driven T cells assays needs more thoroughly be investigated.

The question thus rises whether TSH-R (or other candidate antigen) peptide driven responses of peripheral T cells differ in TGF-β, IL-10, IL-4 and IFN-γ production between Graves' ophthalmopathy patients and healthy controls?

6. FURTHER RESEARCH ON ABNORMALITIES IN THE EFFECTOR PHASE OF THE IMMUNE REACTION

Transfer models of autoreactive T cells and some transgenic animal models have been useful to obtain a better insight in the effector phase. In essence, two major patterns of autoimmune effector reactivity can be discerned: a destructive TH1 pattern of autoreactivity and the development in the affected organ of a local lymphoid tissue that is not necessarily destructive (Fig. 3).

The destructive effector phases of autoimmune endocrinopathies are now generally considered to be largely TH1 mediated. The TH1 mediated destruction of target cells is predominantly reached via the production of γ-IFN by antigen specific CD4[+] and CD8[+] T cells. This cytokine activates macrophages to efficiently kill the target. Such TH1 type of reactivity is best seen in the T cell transfer models of organ-specific autoimmune diseases. Here, autoreactive effector T cells are transferred to susceptible recipients to induce disease, e.g. the transfer of islet-specific diabetogenic clonal T cells to young NOD mice leads to diabetes.[61] The beauty of these models is that they are in fact pure effector phases, since autosensitization was in the donor animals. The lesions in the transfer models are characterized by a simultaneous infiltration in or around the target of T cells, DC and various types of accessory and scavenger macrophages.[62] The latter are found in close opposition to target cells, while T cells are seen in apposition to DC. These data show that DC-T cell interactions also take place in the target tissue during the effector phases. Interestingly, it has been shown that the target cells themselves need not to be recognized by the infiltrating T cells to be actually destroyed.[63] The recognition of the autoantigen by the T cell in the context of the MHC-class II molecules on the APC suffices.

The question thus arises: Is there an intermediate role for antigen-presenting cells in the presumed TH2-fibroblast/adipocyte interaction, or do TH2 cells directly react with fibroblasts/adipocytes?

The excessive production of proinflammatory cytokines, resulting from APC-T cell interactions such as γ-IFN and IL-1, creates a local micromilieu in which certain cells, e.g. insular β cells, are unable to survive and will go into apoptosis due to an excessive NO radical production.[64] Thyrocytes will start to express the Fas molecule under these circumstances of enhanced local cytokine production.[65] The expression of this apoptosis-inducing molecule will contribute to thyroid cell disappearance in the final stages of autoimmune thyroiditis. The latter phenomenon again implicates an active role of the target organ even in the very late stages of the disease, and may explain the observation that in the OS-chicken a 'thyrocyte-susceptibility factor' determines whether thyrocytes are ultimately 'destroyed'. The question thus arises: Do certain cells in the orbit start to express apoptotic molecules due to the local cytokine milieu? If so, how is this regulated?

Beside TH1 like reactions, a special type of focal infiltrate of lymphoid cells can also be found in the target tissues (Fig. 3). These focal infiltrates are often erroneously described as "inflammatory" infiltrates. These infiltrates are, however, histologically clearly distinct from destructive inflammations and in architecture are similar to the mucosa- and bronchus-associated lymphoid tissues. In the Graves' thyroid[66] they are composed of T cell zones with intermingled DC (in this position called interdigitating cells) and at the periphery of the T cell zones there are frequent high endothelial venules (HEVs). A B cell area (sometimes without a germinal center) is often part of the lymphoid structure. Plasma cells radiate from the lymphoid structure into the surrounding parenchyma.[67] Such focal infiltrates can also be found in the retroocular space in Graves' ophthalmopathy.[1] In Hashimoto goiter and in the thyroiditis of the OS chicken focal intrathyroidal lymphoid tissue development may also become very prominent; showing large secondary B cell follicles with germinal centers.[68] Thyroid follicles adjacent to such local lymphoid tissue are often in an advanced stage of decay, and infiltrated with scavenger type macrophages. The development of B cell follicles in such intrathyroidal lymphoid tissue suggests an ongoing affinity maturation of thyroid reactive autoantibodies at this site. Indeed thyroglobulin has been found trapped on the follicular dendritic cells in the B cell follicles. In diabetes the most explicit histological prototype of such lymphoid tissue is encountered in a TCR-transgenic NOD mouse model, in which virtually all naive $CD4^+$ T cells carry a diabetogenic TCR.[69] This mouse develops an impressive peri-insular lymphoid tissue from the age of 2-3 weeks onwards, in the absence, however, of overt diabetes. That overt diabetes does not develop might be related to the fact that in this TCR-transgenic NOD mice, scavenger macrophages are totally absent from the peri-insular lymphoid tissue and the islet environment.[17] Also in another transgenic virus induced mouse diabetes model this local peri-insular lymphoid tissue has been encountered, and a role of DC in its development proven.[69]

With regard to Graves' ophthalmopathy the questions that can be posed are: What is the function of such B cell follicle containing organized lymphoid structures in the retrobulbar space of Graves' ophthalmopathy patients? Do they play a role in high affinity autoantibody production, and/or do they provide a special TH2-like cytokine milieu leading to retrobulbar activation of preadipocytic fibroblasts and muscle swelling?

7. FUTURE RESEARCH ON ENVIRONMENTAL FACTORS IN GRAVES' EYE DISEASE

Of environmental factors, smoking has appeared to be one of the most important factors.[70,71] In the UK, almost 2/3 of Graves' ophthalmopathy patients smoke cigarettes, in contrast to 10-20% of the normal healthy population. The mechanisms behind the association are not clear at all, and questions that remain are:

– Does smoking lead to immune dysregulations akin to alterations seen in inherited forms of endocrine autoimmune disease, as seen in the animal models? Smoking does lead to clear alterations in the DC and MØ function in the lung environment,[72] and to altered production of IL-1 and IL-8.[73] Whether this is reflected in systemic or local monocyte, DC and MØ dysfunction needs to be investigated. There is a recent report on serum IL-1RA levels as predictor for the outcome of radiotherapy in smokers with ophthalmopathy.[74]

– Does smoking perhaps lead to such anoxia in the retrobulbar space,[75] that the mechanisms of Feldon's cat model become operative (see Fig. 4)?

– Does smoking perhaps lead to thyrocyte necrosis or thyroid metabolic abnormalities,[76] processes that might also be driving forces behind a thyroid-specific (TSH-R?) autoimmunization (see Fig. 3)?

Another environmental involves the effect of exogenous retroviruses. These viruses may either dysregulate the function of immune cells, e.g. avian leukosis virus[77] and feline/murine leukemia virus,[78] or induce de novo antigen expression on thyrocytes and fibroblasts. Particular notice should be given here to an earlier observation from the group of Grubeck-Löbenstein and Wick on the rather specific presence in Graves' thyrocytes, Graves' orbital fibroblasts and Graves' orbital fat cells of gag-2 protein-like material of human foamy retrovirus.[79]

8.   FUTURE RESEARCH ON IMMUNE
INTERVENTIONS IN GRAVES' EYE DISEASE

These recent findings open possibilities to embark on new approaches for therapeutic or preventive immune interventions. Particularly the identification of the TSH-R as an important autoantigen, the role of smoking, and the role of certain cytokines in controlling an excessive immune response to self are currently important here.

The transgenically expressed and purified extracellular domain of the TSH-R or peptides of the TSH-R might be used in application of such vaccines in protocols aimed at inducing tolerance. Oral and nasal vaccination which lead to an entry of the autoantigen via the mucosal surface of the airways or gut, may under particular conditions lead to tolerance induction.[80] Will it be possible to induce oral or nasal tolerance using TSH-R peptides in the BALB/C mouse model or cat model of Graves' eye disease?

A very novel approach to induce tolerance is the use of specific types of DC.[81] Some DC, e.g. those from the liver or eye environment or those cultured in the presence of IL-10 or TGF-β, have a superb antigen presenting capability, but they do not stimulate TH1 cells but induce states of anergy/tolerance. Are vaccinations with such DC, when loaded with TSH-R peptides, capable of inducing a state of TSH-R tolerance or even breaking or deviating the state of effector T cell autosensitization? Is perhaps a local treatment in the thyroid or orbit with the immunosuppressive cytokines IL-1 RA, IL-10, or TGF-β sufficient to induce such tolerance?

With regard to smoking it needs to be established whether stopping of smoking improves the outcome of the various immunomodulating regimens presently in use, or whether stopping of smoking is indicated to prevent the development of Graves' disease and Graves' eye disease after radioactive treatment of the thyroid. It goes without saying that careful monitoring of these novel therapeutic approaches needs a further refinement of the methods to score the severity of Graves' eye disease. Also the anatomical structure of the intra-orbital connective tissue need probably to be taken into account here.[82]

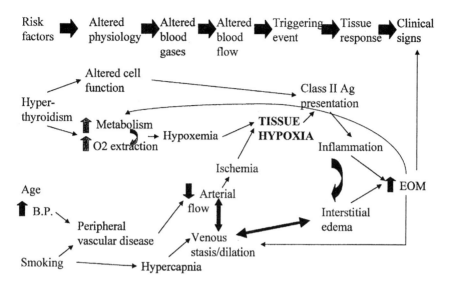

PATHOPHYSIOLOGY OF GRAVES' OPHTHALMOPATHY

Figure 4. The pathophysiology of Graves' ophthalmopathy is multifactorial, involving hormonal, inflammatory, vascular, and mechanical components. The unifying hypothesis described in this figure focuses on the role of tissue hypoxia as the triggering event. The substrate is dependent upon the presence of one or more risk factors, including hyperthyroidism, older age, hypertension, and smoking. Each risk factor contributes to an alteration in normal physiological processes. Hyperthyroidism alters the function of multiple organ and tissue systems and raises the basal metabolic rate leading to an increase in oxygen extraction. It also alters numbers of macrophages in extra-ocular muscles, particularly in the inferior rectus muscle.[83] The other risk factors contribute to onset of peripheral vascular disease. Some of these risk factors contribute to orbital hypoxemia and hypercapnia while others reduce arterial flow, leading to venous stasis. These factors contribute to relative ischemia, producing the tissue hypoxia, central to the model. Inflammation from tissue hypoxia and immune reaction secondary to surface antigen presentation from thyroid-induced alteration of cell function cause interstitial edema in the orbital tissues. This inflammation adds to the interstitial edema associated with venous stasis to promote swelling of the extraocular muscles, pathognomonic of Graves' ophthalmopathy. The isolated orbital compartment is more likely than other regions to foster tissue hypoxia because the extraocular muscles have high metabolic needs and because any increase in tissue swelling decreases venous return, producing a downward spiral of more higher tissue pressure and reduced perfusion of tissues. (Used by permission, Steven Feldon, M.D., copyright 1998, all rights reserved).

ACKNOWLEDGEMENTS
We thank Ms. Geertje de Korte for secretarial assistance. Work in the laboratory of HAD is supported by various grants of NWO, the DFN and the EU.

9. REFERENCES

1. Weetman AP, Cohen S, Gatter KC, Fells P, Shine B. Immunohistochemical analysis of the retrobulbar tissues in Graves' ophthalmopathy. Clin Exp Immunol 1989;75:222-227.
2. Burch H, Wartofsky L. Graves' ophthalmopathy: current concepts regarding pathogenesis and management. Endocr Rev 1993; 14:747-793.
3. Wall JR, Boucher BA, Salvi M, *et al*. Pathogenesis of thyroid associated ophthalmopathy: an autoimmune disorder of the eye muscle associated with Graves' hyperthyroidism and Hashimoto's thyroiditis. Clin Immunol Immunopathol 1993; 68:1-8.
4. Kubota S, Gunji K, Ackrell BAC, Cochran B, Stolarski C, Wengrowicz S, Kennerdell JS, Hiromatsu Y, Wall J. The 64-Kilodalton eye mucle protein is the flavoprotein subunit of mitochondrial succinate dehydrogenase: the corresponding serum antibodies are good markers of an immune-mediated damage to the eye muscle in patients with Graves' hyperthyroidism. J Clin Endocrinol Metab 1998; 83:443-447.
5. Rodbell M. Metabolism of isolated fat cells. I. Effects of hormones on glucose metabolism and lipolysis. J Biol Chem 1964;239:375-380.
6. Rotella CM, Zonefrati R, Toccafondi R, Valente WA, Kohn LD. Ability of monoclonal antibodies to the thyrotropin receptor to increase collagen synthesis in human fibroblasts: an assay which appears to measure exophthalmogenic immunoglobulins in Graves' sera. J Clin Endocrinol Metab 1986; 62:357-67.
7. Crisp MS, Lane C, Halliwell M, Wynford-Thomas D, Ludgate M. Thyrotropin receptor transcripts in human adipose tissue. J Clin Endocrinol Metab 1997; 82:2003-2005.
8. Ludgate M, Crisp M, Lane C, Costagliola S, Vassart G, Weetman A, Daunerie C, Many MC. The thyrotropin receptor in thyroid eye disease. Thyroid 1998; 8:411-413.
9. Bahn RS. Presentation during the VIth International Symposium on Graves' ophthalmopathy, Amsterdam, NL, 27-28, 1998.
10. Sanders J, Oda Y, Roberts SA, Maruyama M, Furmaniak J, Smith BR. Understanding the thyrotropin receptor function-structure relationship. Baillieres Clin Endocrinol Metab 1997;11:451-79.
11. Ludgate M. Presentation during the VIth International Symposium on Graves' ophthalmopathy, Amsterdam, NL, 27-28, 1998.
12. Shimojo N, Kohno Y, Yamaguchi K-I, *et al*. Induction of Graves-like disease in mice by immunization with fibroblasts transfected with the thyrotropin receptor and a class II molecule. Proc Natl Acad Sci USA 1996; 93:11074-11079.
13. Kikuoka S, Shimojo N, Yamaguchi K-I, *et al*. The formation of thyrotropin receptor (TSHR) antibodies in a Graves' animal model requires the N-terminal segment of the TSHR extracellular domain. Endocrinol 1998; 139:1891-1898.
14. Costagliola S, Rodien P, Many MC, Ludgate M, Vassart G. Genetic immunization against the human thyrotropin receptor causes thyroiditis and allows production of monoclonal antibodies recognizing the native receptor. J Immunol 1998;160:1458-65.
15. Lotze MT, Farhood H, Wilson CC, Storkus WJ. Dendritic cell therapy of cancer and HIV infection. In: Lotze MT, Thomson AW, eds. Dendritic cells. Biology and clinical applications. Academic Press, 1999:361-401.
16. Bonifacio E, Christie MR. Islet cell antigens in the prediction and prevention of insulin-dependent diabetes mellitus. Ann Med 1997;29:405-12.
17. Drexhage HA, Delemarre FGA, Radosevic K, Leenen PJM. Dendritic cells in autoimmunity. In: Lotze MT, Thomson AW, eds. Dendritic cells. Biology and clinical applications. Academic Press, 1999:361-401.

18. Many MC, Maniratunga S, Varis I, Dardenne M, Drexhage HA, Denef J-F. Two-step development of Hashimoto-like thyroiditis in genetically autoimmune prone non-obese diabetic mice: effects of iodine-induced cell necrosis. J Endocrinol 1995;147:311-320.

19. Hoek A, Allaerts W, Leenen PJM, Schoemaker J, Drexhage HA. Dendritic cell and macrophages in the pituitary and the gonads. Evidence for their role in the fine regulation of the reproductive endocrine response. Eur J Endocrinol 1997;136:8-24.

20. Allaerts W, Fluitsma DM, Hoefsmit ECM, *et al*. Immunohistochemical morphological and ultrastructural resemblance between dendritic cells and folliculo-stellate cells in normal human and rat anterior pituitaries. J Neuroendocrinol 1996;8:17-29.

21. Simons PJ, Delemarre FGA, Drexhage HA. Antigen-presenting dendritic cells as regulators of the growth of thyrocytes: A role of interleukin-1β and interleukin-6. Endocrinol 1998;139:3148-3156.

22. Gu D, O'Reilly L, Molony L, Cooke A, Sarvetnick N. The role of infiltrating macrophages in islet destruction and regrowth in a transgenic model. 1995;8:483-492.

23. Sundick RS. Target organ defects in thyroid autoimmune disease. Immunol Res 1989;8:39-60.

24. Simons PJ, Delemarre FGA, Jeucken PHM, Drexhage HA. Pre-autoimmune thyroid abnormalities in the biobreeding diabetes-prone (BB-DP) rat. A possible relation with the intrathyroidal accumulation of dendritic cells and the initiation of the thyroid autoimmune response. J Endocrinol 1998; 157: 43-51.

25. Bone AJ, Hitchcock PR, Dunger A. Islet cell cytotoxicity and disease progression in the BB rat. Diabetologia 1997;40, A86 (abstract).

26. Homo-Delarche F, Boitard C. Autoimmune diabetes: the role of the islets of Langerhans. Immunol Today 1996;17:456-460.

27. Robinson CP, Yamamoto H, Peck AB, Humphreys-Beher MG. Genetically programmed development of salivary gland abnormalities in the NOD (nonobese diabetic)-scid mouse in the absence of detectable lymphocytic infiltration: a potential trigger for sialoadenitis of NOD mice. Clin Immunol Immunopathol 1996;79:50-59.

28. Ihm SH, Lee KU, Yoon JW. Studies on autoimmunity for initiation of beta-cells in BB rats. Diabetes 1991;40:269-274.

29. Wilders-Truschnig MM, Drexhage HA, Leb G, *et al*. Chromatographically purified IgG of endemic and sporadic goiter patients sitmulates FRTL-5 cell growth in a mitotoc arrest assay. J Clin Endocrinol Metab 1990; 70:444-452.

30. Bretzel RG, Platzer A, Schaeffer R. Immunopathological findings and thyroid autoantibodies in thyroid autonomy. Acta Med Austriaca 1990;17:20-24.

31. Mooij P, De Wit HJ, Bloot AM, Wilders-Truschnig MM, Drexhage HA. Iodine deficiency induces thyroid autoimmune reactivity in Wistar rats. Endocrinol 1993;133:1197-1204.

32. Wilders-Truschnig MM, Kabel PJ, Drexhage HA, *et al*. Intrathyroidal dendritic cells, epitheloid cells and giant cells in iodine deficient goiter. Am J Pathol 1989; 135:219-225.

33. Markholst H. Characterization of the autosomal recessive T cell lymphopenic trait of DP-BB rats. Exp Clin Endocrinol Diabetes 1997; 105:23.

34. McKeever U, Mordes JP, Greiner DL, *et al*. Adoptive transfer of autoimmune diabetes and thyroiditis to athymic rats. Proc Natl Acad Sci USA 1990;87:7618-7622.

35. Georgiou HM, Lagarde AC, Bellgrau D. T cell dysfunction the the diabetes-prone BB rat. A role for thymic migrants that are not T cell precursos. J Exp Med 1988;167:132-148.

36. Georgiou HM, Constantinou D, Mandel TE. Prevention of autoimmunity in nonobese diabetic (NOD) mice by neonatal transfer of allogeneic thymic macrophages. Autoimmunity 1995;21:89-97.

37. Delemarre FGA, Simons PJ, De Heer HJ, Drexhage HA. Signs of immaturity of splenic dendritic cells from the autoimmune prone biobreeding rat: Consequences for the in vitro expansion of regulator and effector T cells. J Immunol 1999;162:1795-1801.

38. Jansen A, Van Hagen M, Drexhage HA. Defective maturation and function of antigenpresenting cells in type 1 diabetes. Lancet 1995;345:491-492.

39. Takahashi M, Honeyman MC, Harison LC. Defective monocyte-derived dendricit cells from high-risk IDDM relatives. Diabetologia 1997;40:A23 (abstract).

40. Serreze DV, Gaskins HR, Leiter EH. Defects in the differentiation and function fo antigen presenting cells in NOD/Lt mice. J Immunol 1993;150:2534-2543.

41. Badenkoop K, Walfish PG, Rau H, et al. Susceptibility and resistance alleles of human leukocyte antigen (HLA) DQA1 and HLA DQB1 are shared in endocrine autoimmune disease. J Clin Endocrinol Metab 1995; 80:2112-7.

42. Huang W, Connor E, Rosa TD, et al. Although DR3-DQB1*0201 may be associated with multiple component diseases of the autoimmune polyglandular syndromes, the human leukocyte antigen DR4-DQB1*0302 haplotype is implicated only in beta-cell autoimmunity. J Clin Endocrinol Metab 1996; 81:2559-63.

43. Yanagawa T, Hidaka Y, Guimaraes V, Soliman M, DeGroot LJ. CTLA-4 gene polymorphism associated with Graves' disease in Caucasian population. J Clin Endocrinol Metab 1995; 80:41-5.

44. Kotsa K, Watson PF, Weetman AP. A CTLA-4 gene polymorphism is associated with both Graves disease and autoimmune hypothyroidism. Clin Endocrinol 1997; 46:551-554.

45. Kabel PJ, Voorbij HAM, De Haan M, Van der Gaag RD, Drexhage HA. Intrathyoroidal dendritic cells in Graves' disease and simple goitre. J Clin Endocrinol Metab 1988; 65:199-207.

46. Nygaard B, Faber J, Hegedüs L, Mølholm Hansen J. [131]I treatment of nodular non-toxic goitre. Eur J Endocrinol 1996;134:15-20.

47. Hirsch C, Spyra JL, Langhammer HR, Laubenbacher C, Senekowitsch-Schmidtke R, Schwaiger M. Occurrence of immune hyperthyroidism after radioiodine therapy of autonomous goiter. Med Klin 1997; 92:130-7.

48. Saber E, McDonnell J, Zimmermann KM, Yugar JE, Feldon SE. Extraocular muscle changes in experimental orbital venous stasis: some similarities to Graves' orbitopathy. Graefes Arch Clin Exp Ophthalmol 1996; 234:331-6.

49. Davies C, Troy GC. Deep mycotic infections in cats. J Am Anim Hosp Assoc 1996;32:380-91.

50. Kraemer MH, Donadi EA, Tambascia MA, Magna LA, Prigenzi LS. Relationship between HLA antigens and infectious agents in contributing towards the development of Graves' disease. Immunol Invest 1998;27:17-29.

51. Wenzel BE, Peters A, Zubaschev I. Bacterial virulence antigens and the pathogenesis of autoimmune thyroid diseases (AITD). Exp Clin Endocrinol Diabetes. 1996;104:74-8.

52. Cohen SB, Weetman AP. Characterization of different types of experimental autoimmune thyroiditis in the Buffalo strain rat. Clin Exp Immunol 1987;69:25-32.

53. Tas MPR, De Haan-Meulman M, Kabel PJ, Drexhage HA. Defects in monocyte polarization and dendritic cell clustering in patients with Graves disease. A putative role of a nonspecific immunoregulatory factor related to retroviral p15E. Clin Endocrinol 1991; 34:441-448.

54. Mühlberg T, Spitzweg Ch, Heberling H-J, Heufelder AE. Regulation of interleukin-1 receptor antagonist gene and protein variants by ionizing irradiation in Graves' retroocular fibroblasts. VIth International Symposium on Graves' ophthalmopathy. Amsterdam, November 27-28, 1998.

55. Wakelkamp IMMJ, Gerding MN, Van der Meer JWC, Prummel MF, Wiersinga WM. Serum cytokines are elevated in Graves' ophthalmopathy. VIth International Symposium on Graves' ophthalmopathy. Amsterdam, November 27-28, 1998.

56. Barbesino G, Tomer Y, Concepcion ES, Davies TF, Greenberg DA. Linkage analysis of candidate genes in autoimmune thyroid disease. II. Selected gender-related genes and the X-chromosome. International consortium for the genetics of autoimmune thyroid disease. J Clin Endocrinol Metab 1998; 83:3290-5.

57. Grubeck-Loebenstein B, Trieb K, Sztankay A, Holter W, Anderl H, Wick G. Retrobulbar T cells from patients with Graves' ophthalmopathy are CD8[+] and specifically recognize autologous fibroblasts. J Clin Invest 1994;93:2738-2743.

58. Förster G, Otto E, Hansen C, Ochs K, Kahaly G. Analysis of orbital T cells in thyroid-associated ophthalmopathy. Clin Exp Immunol 1998;112:427-434.

59. Pappa A, Calder V, Ajjan R, Fells P, Ludgate M, Weetman AP, Lightman S. Analysis of extraocular muscle-infiltrating T cells in thyroid-associated ophthalmopathy (TAO). Clin Exp Immunol 1997;109:362-369.

60. Heufelder AE. T-cell restriction in thyroid eye disease. Thyroid 1998; 8:419-22.

61. Bergman B, Haskins K. Autoreactive T cell clones from the nonobese diabetic mouse. Proc Soc Exp Biol Med 1997; 214:41-48.

62. Rosmalen JGM, Martin T, Voerman JSA, Drexhage HA, Haskins K, Leenen PJM. Dual role for dendritic cells and macrophages in diabetes development: initiation of infiltration and initiations of destruction. Submitted.

63. Lo D, Reilly C, Marconi LA, *et al*. Regulation of CD4 T cell reactivity to self and non-self. Int Rev Immunol 1995; 13:147-160.

64. Eizirik DL, Leijerstam F. The inducible form of nitric oxide synthase (iNOS) in insulinproducing cells (Review). Diabetes Metab 1994; 20:116-122.

65. Mitsiades N, Poulaki V, Kotoula V, *et al*. Fas/Fas ligand up-regulation and BCL-2 down-regulation may be significant in the pathogenesis of Hashimoto's thyroiditis. J Clin Endocrinol Metab 1998; 83:2199-2203.

66. Kabel PJ, Voorbij HAM, De Haan-Meulman M, Pals ST, Drexhage HA. High endothelial venules present in lymphoid cell accumulations in thyroid affected by autoimmune disease. A study in men and BB rat of functional activity and development. J Clin Endocrinol Metab 1989; 68:744-751.

67. Drexhage HA. Dendritic cells and class II MHC expression on thyrocytes during the autoimmune thyroid disease of the BB rat. Clin Immunol Immunopathol 1990; 55:9-22.

68. Wick G, Hu Y, Schwarz S, Kroemer G. Immunoendocrine communication via the hypothalamo-pituitary-adrenal axis in autoimmune diseases. Endocr Rev 1993; 14:539-563.

69. Ludewig B, Odermatt B, Landmann S, Hengartner H, Zinkernagel RM. Dendritic cells induce autoimmune diabetes and maintain disease via de novo formation of local lymphoid tissue. J Exp Med 1998; 188:1493-1501.

70. Shine B, Fells P, Edwards OM, Weetman AP. Association between Graves' ophthalmopathy and smoking. Lancet 1990; 335:1261-3.

71. Prummel MF, Wiersinga WM. Smoking and risk of Graves' disease. JAMA 1993; 269:479-482.

72. Van Haarst JM, Hoogsteden HC, De Wit HJ, Verhoeven GT, Havenith CE, Drexhage HA. Dendritic cells and their precursors isolated from human bronchoalveolar lavage: immunocytologic and functional properties. Am J Respir Cell Mol Biol 1994; 11:344-350.

73. Kuschner WG, D'Alessandro A, Wong H, Blanc PD. Dose-dependent cigarette smoking-related inflammatory responses in healthy adults. Eur Respir J 1996;9:1989-94.

74. Hofbauer LC, Mohlberg T, Konig A, Heufelder G, Schworm H-D, Heufelder AE. Soluble interleukin-1 receptor antagonist serum levels in smokers and nonsmokers with Graves' ophthalmopathy undergoing orbital radiotherapy. J Clin Endocrinol Metab 1997; 82:2244-2247.

75. Metcalfe RA, Weetman AP. Stimulation of extraocular muscle fibroblasts by cytokines and hypoxia: possible role in thyroid-associated ophthalmopathy. Clin Endocrinol 1994; 40:67-72.

76. Colzani R, Fang SL, Alex S, Braverman LE. The effect of nicotine on thyroid function in rats. Metabolism 1998;47: 154-7.

77. Carter JK, Smith RE. Rapid induction of hypothyroidism by an avian leukosis virus. Infect Immun 1983; 40:795-805.

78. Good RA, Ogasaware M, Liu WT, Lorenz E, Day NK. Immunosuppressive actions of retroviruses. Lymphology 1990; 23:56-9.

79. Wick G, Trieb K, Aguzzi A, Recheis H, Ander H, Grubeck-Loebenstein B. Possible role of human foamy virus in Graves' disease. Intervirology 1993; 35:101-107.

80. Strober W, Kelsall B, Marth T. Oral tolerance. J Clin Immunol 1998; 18:1-30.

81. Lu L, Khoury SJ, Sayegh MH, Thomson AW. Dendritic cell tolerogenicity and prespects for dendritic cell-based therapy of allograft rejection and autoimmunity. In: Lotze MT, Thomson AW, eds. Dendritic cells. Biology and clinical applications. Academic Press, 1999:361-401.

82. Koornneef L, Donné Schmidt E, van der Gaag R. The orbit: structure, autoantigens, and pathology. In: Wall JR, How J, eds. Current Issues in Endocrinology and Metabolism: Graves' Ophthalmopathy. Oxford: Blackwell Scientific Publications, 1990:1-16.

83. Schmidt ED, van Hogerwou G, van der Gaag R, Wiersinga WM, Asmussen G, Koornneef L. Site-dependent effects of experimental hypo- and hyperthyroidism on resident macrophages in extraocular muscles of rats: a quantitative immunohistochemical study. J Endocrinol 1992; 135:485-493.

Index

Additional Permissions Information

Chapter 4, Figure 2, page 60: Reproduced with permission from Brown M. Dobyns. Present concepts of the pathologic physiology of exophtalmos. Journal of Endocrinology and Metabolism 1950; 10: 1202-1230. © The Endocrine Society